YOGA GEMS

YOGA GEMS

Georg Feuerstein

BANTAM BOOKS

NEW YORK   TORONTO   LONDON   SYDNEY   AUCKLAND

YOGA GEMS

PUBLISHING HISTORY
Bantam trade paperback / April 2002

Book design by Joseph Rutt

Library of Congress Cataloging-in-Publication Data
Feuerstein, Georg.
    Yoga gems / Georg Feuerstein.
        p. cm.
    Includes bibliographical references.
    ISBN 0-553-38088-5
        1. Yoga, Haòha.   I. Title.

RA781.7 .F484 2001
613.7′046—dc21   2001043699

Published simultaneously in the United States and Canada

Bantam Books are published by Bantam Books, a division of Random
House, Inc. Its trademark, consisting of the words "Bantam Books" and
the portrayal of a rooster, is Registered in U.S. Patent and Trademark Of-
fice and in other countries. Marca Registrada. Bantam Books, 1540 Broad-
way, New York, New York 10036.

PRINTED IN THE UNITED STATES OF AMERICA

RRH 10 9 8 7 6 5 4 3 2 1

ANCIENT INVOCATION

From the unreal lead me to the Real.
From darkness lead me to Light.
From death lead me to Immortality.

—BRIHAD-ARANYAKA-UPANISHAD

FOR LAWRENCE AND HILLARY

"Dream abides. It is the only thing that abides; vision abides."

—MIGUEL DE UNAMUNO

CONTENTS

PREFACE

This book is intended for the tens of millions of Yoga practitioners around the world, for those many millions more who are curious about Yoga, and for those countless others who simply seek intelligent inspiration and encouragement in their daily life.

While the current wave of Yoga focuses on its value as a physical discipline for fitness and stress reduction, many people are cognizant of Yoga's psychological and spiritual potency as well. With Baby Boomers reaching the critical midlife period, which many psychologists recognize as a time for overall lifestyle and spiritual reappraisal, Yoga's future as a tradition of wisdom and core spiritual values is assured. Yoga's five-thousand-year-old heritage contains incredible nuggets of spiritual and psychological insight, which *Yoga Gems* seeks to make available through simple but profound quotations.

I have focused on the wisdom of modern Yoga masters, who speak our language more closely, but I have also drawn from the teachings of the ancient sages. In some cases, when there was no name attached to a particular piece of wisdom, I have cited the textual source. Traditional sources quoted from in this compilation include works written in Sanskrit, Pali, Tibetan, Prakrit, Marathi, Tamil, and English. They reflect the Yoga traditions of Hinduism, Buddhism, and Jainism. These three world religions—which are really whole cultures—have Yoga for their essence.

There are also many quotes from contemporary adepts from the Hindu and Buddhist Yoga traditions. In addition, I have selected poignant quotes from a few individuals who would not call themselves adepts but who practice Yoga and have expressed their thoughts about Yoga particularly well.

Yoga has produced a galaxy of extraordinary individuals who were not only spiritual giants but also philosophical and/or literary geniuses. As a professional Indologist, I have access to many of the traditional sources and have translated a good many Sanskrit texts into English. Few days go by when I don't read a passage or two from one of my favorite Hindu or Buddhist Yoga scriptures for my enjoyment and spiritual upliftment. As a practitioner and teacher for over thirty years, I have also become very familiar with the needs of ordinary people trying to make sense of life and Yoga.

Each page in *Yoga Gems* features one or more authoritative quotations of practical wisdom that has been selected because it may touch your heart, inspire your spiritual life, or stimulate your thinking about deeper matters. Themes include the value of silence; how to meditate; golden rules for living; how to infuse life with joy; creating hope; the importance of thinking positively; universal kinship; seeing the larger picture; overcoming suffering; dealing with grief, loss, anger, and jealousy; remembering one's true inner self; cultivating the good; developing self-discipline; the nature of love; cultivating patience, inner growth, caring, and so on.

"There is nothing more powerful than Yoga," declares one medieval Sanskrit text. I hope that the sayings, poems, and anecdotes gathered here will convey something of the truth behind this claim. Ultimately, however, the proof of the pudding is in the eating. May this volume inspire you to explore the heritage of Yoga personally and practically. Having myself benefited from Yoga's versatile teachings over the past thirty-five years, I can guarantee that you will not be disappointed.

—GEORG FEUERSTEIN
Yoga Research and Education Center
2400A County Center Drive
Santa Rosa, CA 95403
www.yrec.org

ACKNOWLEDGMENTS

My profound gratitude goes to the masters who have been guiding my life. Their presence has brought me wisdom, beauty, direction, and also challenge.

As always, my wife and spiritual partner Trisha Lamb Feuerstein has had a hand in the making of this volume. My love and gratitude go to her for her steadfast commitment, caring, and far-too-long hours of work.

My heartfelt thanks go to Wolfgang Saumweber, whose friendship, kindness, and generosity have helped my work significantly.

I would also like to cordially thank my literary agent, Carol Susan Roth, who unfailingly champions my writings and seems to have no doubt that one day I will write that top-ten bestseller. I will keep trying against all the odds, just for her.

Many thanks to Toni Burbank, senior editor at Bantam, for seeing the potential of this book and paying me for doing what I most enjoy: being in the company of great masters and their inspiring ideas and ideals. And kind thanks to the other good spirits at Bantam.

INTRODUCTION

WHAT IS YOGA?

It is impossible to give a precise answer to this simple question, mainly because Yoga is so incredibly comprehensive and encompasses such a tremendous variety of approaches. The word itself, which stems from the ancient Sanskrit language, means both "union" and "discipline." Thus *yoga* conveys "unitive spiritual discipline" or "the spiritual discipline of integration." What the tradition of Yoga seeks to integrate is head and heart, as well as psyche and world, on the basis of a profound spiritual realization that transcends head, heart, psyche, and world.

That realization is variously called *Self-realization, God-realization, enlightenment,* or *liberation.* It consists in discovering a marvelous truth about ourselves: We are not merely a particular body, mind, or personality, but the very foundation of *all* bodies, minds, and personalities—in fact, of all animate and inanimate things in the universe. The great masters of Yoga insist that we are first and foremost the One Being that is the ultimate substance of the universe. And that substance is pure Consciousness. What a vision of our human potential!

The masters of Yoga arrived at their insights about Oneness not through mere fanciful speculation but through direct realization. Yoga has from the beginning been intensively experiential and even experimental. Acknowledging Yoga's extraordinary heritage, Carl Gustav Jung remarked that it is "one of the greatest things the human mind has ever created."

Yoga is the art of fashioning the alabaster block of our body-mind into a beautiful lucid sculpture that reflects the Light of the ultimate, singular Being, which is eternally blissful and supreme conscious. To practice Yoga, we must become craftsmen and -women of great skill and sensitivity. We master the art of Yoga as we gain self-knowledge and the capacity for self-transcendence. Searching deep into our mind and heart, we learn to exceed our ordinary boundaries and discover that we are immeasurably vast, surpassing even Nature itself. We realize that Nature, grand and fascinating as it is, is only a temporary aspect of the ultimate One, which transcends space and time.

THE QUEST FOR HAPPINESS

Yoga provides convincing answers to the Big Questions—Who am I? What must I do? What is the purpose of life? and so on. Basically, the human enterprise can be looked at as a diversified quest for happiness. We all want happiness, but frequently or perhaps even typically we look for it in the wrong places. We settle instead for temporary pleasures ("fun"), not understanding that pleasure is the obverse side of pain. Our lives thus are often characterized not by happiness (*ananda*) but by suffering (*duhkha*). Yoga digs deep into the reasons for this failure to tap into lasting happiness and shows us how to change our self-sabotaging behavior. It all begins and ends with the complex human mind, which is governed by ignorance and any number of negative emotions. Yoga not only points the way out of the maze our mind tends to create but provides concrete practical means for doing so.

Yoga contains all kinds of theoretical considerations, but these are integrally connected with practical steps for overcoming suffering and attaining abiding happiness through inner freedom. Looking only at the physical side of existence, neurophysiologists tell us that happiness depends on the free and harmonious flow of neuropeptides. This perspective helps us begin to appreciate that body and mind are a working team and therefore need to be kept in optimal condition.

Happiness, however, is not merely a brain function or mental state. It is who or what we are when our mental confusion is lifted and we have recovered our true Identity—as the Spirit. Happiness, or bliss, is of the nature of our spiritual Identity—the so-called transcendental Self. What we normally experience as happiness is merely a physiological-mental reflection of that deeper happiness, which can never be taken away from us. It is our true Self. This is the central message of all branches and schools of Yoga.

A GLIMPSE AT THE HISTORY OF YOGA

Given Yoga's protracted history, which has been shaped by at least two hundred generations of practitioners, we are justified in expecting a great deal of practical wisdom from it.

Yoga dates back to the Indus-Sarasvati civilization, which flourished c. 3000 B.C.E. but whose historical roots lie still further back in time. In fact, avant-garde scholarship has recognized the Indic civilization to be the oldest continuous civilization on Earth, with towns like Mehrgarh now being assigned to the seventh millennium B.C.E.

The earliest evidence of yogic ideas and practices can be found in the *Rig-Veda*, a collection of over a thousand sacred hymns composed in archaic Sanskrit. For thousands of years, this hymnody was faithfully transmitted by oral tradition—so faithfully, in fact, that the available recensions differ by only a single syllable.

At that early time, Yoga was still intimately connected with the sacrificial rituals of the Vedic people. Subsequently, Yoga was pursued as "inner sacrifice": a multipronged discipline of focusing the mind upon the transcendental Spirit, or One Being, while letting go of all inessential things. This led to a growing movement of radical world renunciation that produced, for instance, Buddhism and Jainism. Many Yoga masters, however, acknowledged early on that dispassion need not result in flight from the world.

One of the most remarkable Yoga scriptures to teach an integrative path of inner renunciation combined with engaging the world and fulfilling one's obligations is the *Bhagavad-Gita* ("Lord's Song"). This beautiful work, which Mahatma Gandhi called "My Mother," was probably authored in its present form around 400–500 B.C.E. It combines Karma-Yoga ("discipline of self-transcending action"), Bhakti-Yoga ("discipline of devotional surrender to the Divine"), and Jnana-Yoga ("discipline of wise discrimination between the real and the unreal").

Yoga assumed its classical form around 200 C.E. under Patanjali, the compiler of the *Yoga-Sutra* ("Aphorisms of Yoga"). His well-known eightfold path consists of moral discipline, self-restraint, posture, breath control, sensory inhibition, concentration, meditation, and ecstasy. The goal, as with any form of Yoga, is spiritual realization or liberation.

Hatha-Yoga ("forceful discipline"), the most popular yogic approach in modern times, sprang up around 1000 C.E. It is best known for its numerous bodily postures, which are designed to maintain or restore health and enhance physical vitality. The underlying idea is that the human body is very precious, because it serves as the foundation for spiritual realization. Traditional Hatha-Yoga even seeks to transform the body into a transubstantiated or "divine body" that can withstand the ravages of time and is equipped with all kinds of extraordinary capacities. Much of contemporary Hatha-Yoga, by contrast, revolves around physical fitness and health, whereas traditional Yoga is chiefly about mental health and actualizing our full spiritual potential.

Other traditional yogic approaches include Mantra-Yoga, consisting in the recitation of potent sounds (such as the sacred syllable *om*); Tantra-Yoga, consisting in extensive ritual practices and elaborate meditative visualizations (this approach is often misinterpreted by Westerners as a form of spiritualized sexuality); and Laya-Yoga ("discipline of meditative absorption"), consisting in practices that endeavor to awaken the "serpent power," or *kundalini,* which is the universal energy as it manifests in a limited way in the human body.

Yoga made its tentative entry into the modern Western world in 1785 with the first English translation of the *Bhagavad-Gita*. Then, at the World Parliament of Religions, held in Chicago in 1893, Swami Vivekananda brought Yoga to the attention of a much wider audience. Since then, many more Indian Yoga initiates and masters have brought the wisdom of Yoga to the West. Over the millennia, Yoga has continued to develop in response to changing social and cultural conditions. Today, it is being adapted to the needs of its tens of millions of Western practitioners. The popularization of Yoga has led to a certain amount of oversimplification and distortion, yet in the hearts of its genuine practitioners, Yoga's torch of wisdom burns as brightly as ever. We can expect it to light our path into the future, but for this we need to actually practice it. Yoga cannot unlock our immense spiritual and creative potential unless we practice it steadfastly. If this book inspires you to do so, it will have fulfilled its purpose.

May your path be blessed with growth and higher realizations.

I
MIND—MAKER
OF DESTINY

ॐ

The human mind is a wondrous thing. It can create disease or heal us. It can hurl us into hell (suffering) or elevate us into heaven (happiness).

If we look at life closely, with a mind free from preconceptions and delusions, we quickly realize our days are filled with experiences that can be summed up in one word: *suffering*. As long as we look at life through the rose-colored glasses of wishful thinking and pretense, however, we are bound to tell ourselves and others that, in the words of Voltaire, this is the best of all possible worlds.

In contrast, the Indian sages have always been realistic in their assessment of human existence and the world as a whole. Apart from some fleeting moments of pleasure, which must not be confused with real happiness, ours is not an enviable lot.

This wisdom of the ancient Indian sages was given exquisite expression by the enlightened master Gautama, later to be known as "the Buddha" or "Awakened One." Like many of the sages remembered in history, Gautama was born into a royal family, but he abandoned his comfortable court life at the age of twenty-nine to take up the most challenging yogic practices. Six years later, after many years of exploring the dead end of severe asceticism, he opted for the middle path by restoring his physical well-being and mental balance. In a single night of concentrated self-inquiry, leading him to ever-higher states of consciousness, he attained full enlightenment. He felt moved to share the path he had discovered with others, and in his very first sermon he explained: "Life is suffering; suffering results from egoic desire which is rooted in spiritual ignorance; the elimination of egoic desire and thus of spiritual ignorance brings the end of suffering; the way of terminating egoic desire and spiritual ignorance is the noble eightfold path." The eightfold path consists of right view, right resolve, right speech, right action, right livelihood, right effort, right mindfulness, and right concentration, and leads to the extinction of suffering.

Gautama arrived at this penetrating insight because he clearly saw that everything is impermanent and lacking a stable center (or "self" or "ego"). Hundreds of great sages before and after him have testified to the same truth; yet we continue to behave as if our life lasts forever and as if everything revolves around us—the ego-personality. As long as we cling to these mistaken notions, we set ourselves up for suffering.

We must not, however, confuse suffering with pain. Our body, for instance, may be in great condition, but we may still be suffering. Conversely, we may have a piercing toothache but not suffer at all. Suffering is something we place on top of pain, and it is also something that, on closer inspection, lies hidden within pleasure. At root, we all know that however great our pleasure may be, it is still limited and cannot last.

The Sanskrit word for suffering is *duhkha*, which means literally "bad axle hole." With a bad or warped axle hole, the wheel will not turn smoothly. The word *duhkha* also can be translated as "bad space." When we are out of touch with our higher nature, we are indeed in bad space, and whether we are in or out of touch is all a matter of the mind.

Although the Yoga masters are very sensitive to the omnipresence of suffering, they are not pessimists. On the contrary, you might call them the greatest optimists alive, for they firmly believe that *all* suffering can be completely overcome. That is, in fact, the purpose of Yoga. The very possibility of suffering is perfectly eliminated through enlightenment. And enlightenment occurs when we discover our true Identity—the eternal, supraconscious Self. As I noted at the beginning of this introduction, whether we enjoy enlightenment or endure bondage is a matter of mind. As the *Amrita-Bindu-Upanishad,* a medieval Sanskrit text, states:

> The mind alone is the cause of bondage and liberation for human beings. Attached to things, it leads to bondage. Emptied of things, it is deemed to lead to liberation.

Bondage means being bound by fear, anger, lust, jealousy, competitiveness, and all the other negative emotions and desires that drive so much of our conventional lives. It stands for psychological limitation or conditioning, which is caused by spiritual ignorance.

Liberation, by contrast, is caused by spiritual knowledge, or wisdom. It consists in enjoying freedom *from* our psychological conditioning in all circumstances, leaving us free *for* intelligent, compassionate activity. Yoga helps us overcome our psychological limitations and thus allows us to recover our innermost spiritual nature, the higher Self, which is eternally free and blissful.

As Swami Muktananda, a great modern master of Siddha-Yoga, once said, "You should welcome heartily the beneficent grace of the mind," for it is the restless mind that starts you on your spiritual journey. It is also the mind, once mastered, that reveals the treasure locked away inside it: our higher, spiritual nature. That higher nature is variously called "transcendental Self," "Spirit," "God," "Lord," "Supreme Being," "ultimate Reality," or "Nirvana."

TO GROW OR NOT TO GROW

๑

Growing is the most important and essential endeavor that a human being can undertake. You can make and lose money; you can be promoted and demoted in the world. Never, at any stage, is there any certainty about what will happen to you in this life. However, there is one thing that nobody can ever take away from you—the growth you attain through your own search for Self-knowledge. Furthermore, this growth and understanding become the foundation that sustains you through any and all worldly difficulties, and that allows you—whatever the form of your physical experience—to find in life a continuously unbroken flow of total well-being.

—SWAMI CHETANANANDA

BECOMING HUMAN

✦

If we are honest with ourselves we see that we are not yet real human beings, not yet truly humane, compassionate, or sensitive creatures. We are not yet independent, aware, intelligent, mature, and responsible, with a concern for all life. Our basic values stem from the self-image—pleasure, power, wealth, and so on. They are the values of the self-focused mind trapped in its desires. We may refine this basic immaturity of the mind, make its indulgences more benevolent, its prejudices more tolerant, but at the core it persists.

—DAVID FRAWLEY

LIFE IS PRECIOUS

꒰

We must never forget that our life is like a paper bag that a few drops of water could destroy. It is like a piece of thin glass that a little gust of wind could shatter. It is like a goatskin filled with air floating on a river, which would sink to the bottom if the air should go out of it. It is like a wall of sand that may collapse at any moment. Therefore, do not merely build castles in the air, but start building them on the ground. Every breath is precious, for once lost it can never return. Make hay while the sun shines. Take advantage of this human body so long as it lasts in searching for the One without whom the entire world is going adrift and astray.

The human form is an invaluable gift. We should avail ourselves of it for the purpose for which it is granted to us. Wife and children, food and drink, we have had in every life. The uniqueness of the human form consists in its ability to realize God as long as it is activated by life. Towards this end we must bend all our energies. This is our real work. The rest is all to no purpose.

—MAHARAJ CHARAN SINGH

YOU BECOME WHAT YOU THINK

❧

As is one's thought, so one becomes. This is an eternal mystery.

—*MAITRI-UPANISHAD*

BE CAREFUL WHAT YOU THINK

❧

One day, an employee of a refrigeration company was accidentally locked up in the ice chamber of a freight train with a temperature of forty degrees below zero. No one heard his shouts for help. He was absolutely terrified and left a record of his suffering scribbled on the walls of the wagon. By the time the train arrived at its destination he had died. Significantly, his death was due not to exposure to subzero temperature but sheer fright, because on that day the refrigeration was not switched on at all. Such is the fate of those who allow their thoughts to be imprisoned in a cold, dark chamber.

—SRI ANANDA ACHARYA

MENTAL SUGGESTION

The mind is susceptible to suggestions. It learns whatever you teach it. If through discrimination you can impress upon it the joy and fullness of life in the spirit and the folly of worldly attachments, then your mind will devote itself more and more to God.

—SWAMI BRAHMANANDA

MENTAL POWER

Fickleness is the very nature of the mind. But if it is endowed with indifference to worldly things and guided toward yogic discipline, it can be steadied in due course. The reason is that there is a power in the mind that, once it becomes interested in something, it quickly develops a fondness for it. Therefore you should coax your mind and create in it a liking for the bliss of the Self.

—JNANADEVA

CONTROLLING THE BRAIN

❧

This cerebral system will ruin you, unless consciously you learn to free yourself from it. This secondary powerhouse continually not only spends energy, but damnably interferes with the very creation of energy in the body.

—PUNDIT ACHARYA

MIND CONTROL

❧

You can learn to control your mind very well—because it is yours, but do not try to control the minds of others and make them dependent. When one becomes dependent, one suffers, so you should learn to be independent, and you should not make others dependent upon you.

—SWAMI RAMA

MENTAL PURITY

❧

You are the master of your mind, and you have to keep it pure.
Your responsibility ends there, the rest is God's business.

—SWAMI VIJNANANANDA

THOUGHT AND ADDICTION

❧

We have many addictions, which we may call habits and inter-
ests, or even skills and talents. Such addictions as drugs, alco-
hol or gambling are but the most evident forms of the
addictive pattern of our entire behavior. Some of us are ad-
dicted to sex, others to food, others to business, knowledge, or
even religious practices. Whatever we become dependent on to
occupy our time or fill our minds is an addiction. All external
seeking—whether for pleasure, wealth, status or knowledge—is
not essentially different than the alcoholic looking for a drink.

Thought is our most basic addiction and from it other
addictions derive like branches. Thought is a habit, an unconscious mechanism of the mind. If you do not believe this,
then try to control your thoughts, try to stop thinking. Obviously thought is not a conscious process but a compulsion. As long as we are ruled by thought we are addicts and
our addiction must distort our perception of reality.

—DAVID FRAWLEY

CHOOSE A SUBLIME IDEAL

❧

If you dedicate yourself to a sublime ideal, your life will continually grow in richness, strength and intensity. It is like a capital investment: you place your capital in a Heavenly bank so that, instead of deteriorating or going to waste, it increases and makes you richer.

—OMRAAM MIKHAËL AÏVANHOV

MAKING LIFE MEANINGFUL

❧

Whether life in itself has a meaning or not: it is up to us to *give* it a meaning. In the hands of an inspired artist a worthless lump of clay turns into a priceless work of art. Why should we not likewise try to make something worthwhile out of the common clay of our lives, instead of lamenting about its worthlessness?

—LAMA ANAGARIKA GOVINDA

RIGHT UNDERSTANDING

෨

Just as one comes to ruin
Through wrong eating and obtains
Long life, freedom from disease,
Strength and pleasure through right eating,

So one comes to ruin
Through wrong understanding
But gains bliss and complete enlightenment
Through right understanding.

—NAGARJUNA

RIGHT VIEW

Right view is vital to the intelligent pursuit of happiness. We are not talking about right view in terms of one person's or one group's views being superior to another's. Right view refers to the harmony of the knowing mind with the nature of phenomena as they actually are. How we view the world shapes how we act and feel in it. If we view the cosmos as personally hostile towards us, or disappointing, or meaningless, we are bound to be haunted by an anxiety which lurks in the dark recesses of our minds and periodically erupts into consciousness with disabling intensity. If we view existence as benevolent or at least benign, it is easier for us to relax into it; we might be more tolerant, more grateful, more gracious, and less inclined to be thrown off balance into the pain of negative emotions.

—RON LEIFER

FROM IGNORANCE TO KNOWLEDGE

❧

One must know that one is ignorant before one can begin to know.

—SRI AUROBINDO

THE MILK OF WISDOM

❧

Like butter hidden in milk,
wisdom dwells in all living beings.
With the mind as the churning rod,
one should ever churn out
wisdom from within oneself.

—*BRAHMA-BINDU-UPANISHAD*

TWO KINDS OF DOUBT

꒳

"Is it wrong to doubt? I don't like to believe blindly," a student said. The Master replied:

"There are two kinds of doubt: destructive and constructive. Destructive doubt is habitual skepticism. Men who cultivate that attitude disbelieve blindly; they shun the work of impartial investigation. Skepticism is a static on one's mental radio that causes him to lose the program of truth.

"Constructive doubt is intelligent questioning and fair examination. Those who cultivate that attitude do not prejudge matters or accept as valid the opinions of others. In the spiritual path, constructive doubters base their conclusions on tests and personal experience: the proper approach to truth."

—PARAMAHANSA YOGANANDA

THE LIMITS OF REASON

꒳

Reason is a finite instrument. It cannot explain many mysterious problems of life. Those who are free from the so-called rationalism and skepticism can march in the path of God-realization.

—SWAMI SIVANANDA SARASWATI

MENTAL CLOUDS

Doubts, like clouds, sail on the mental horizon occasionally. They can be dark and heavy or small and wispy. Sometimes they disappear, but often return unnoticed because of an influx of new experiences. . . . Impatience and restlessness create doubt, but the aspirant is warned that both prevent certain spiritual powers from developing. Remember that impatience is an expression of arrogance of some sort which, if allowed to linger, will undermine faith, hope, and will, and only strengthen the moods of depression. Arrogance is of the ego and is therefore destructive.

—SWAMI SIVANANDA RADHA

FAITH

Faith is the greatest asset of the disciple. If you have faith, you have everything; without faith, you have nothing. Faith is not a result of external observances, it comes by constant inner awareness, not of the sense or the turbulence and disturbances of the mind, but of the soul. . . . As you go deeper within and face the inner light, you become faithful. Where there is faith, there is power and enlightenment.

A disciple lives by faith.

—SWAMI SATYASANGANANDA SARASWATI

THE MIND MUST BE AWAKENED

٭

The mind of ours which is absorbed in deep slumber has to be awakened, for the only obstacle that hinders the soul from merging in the Lord is our mind. The soul is of the essence of the Lord. It is a ray of the divine sun, a spark from the Supreme Being, a drop of the divine ocean. But entangled in the closely woven net of illusion (Maya), it has taken to the company of the mind. The mind itself is in the hands of the senses and is being constantly dragged by them in different directions. The result is that the soul, which is intrinsically pure and sublime, gathers coats of dirt and rust which cover its refulgence.

Both mind and soul feel forlorn and unhappy. They are foreign to this land and have a natural inclination to go back to their source. So long as the mind does not return to its source . . . it does not free the soul. The latter remains powerless to realize its sublime nature and yearns in vain to go back to its home.

—MAHARAJ CHARAN SINGH

FOOLS AND SAGES

٭

Fools are asleep; sages are always awake.

—VARDHAMANA MAHAVIRA

THE SECRET OF PROPER
DISCERNMENT

❧

Yoga never demands the sacrifice of our reason. It only bids us: use it a thousand times more. Yoga does not require us to give up our active lives. It says simply: act, but know *how* to act. Yoga does not by any means wish us to push our understanding aside. It only tells us: discriminate correctly and act fearlessly. Yoga does not expect us to flee from the world and to retire into the Himalayas. It assures us: the refuge you seek you will never find in the outside world. It is within you. Leave the stormy world of the senses behind you, raise your consciousness to the central point of your being and realize that here alone is the force, here alone is the peace and here alone the refuge you are seeking. Yoga teaches us: do not condemn the world. Deify the world by your deeds, purify the world by your utterances and ennoble the world by your presence.

—SELVARAJAN YESUDIAN

PERFECT MIND, PERFECT HEART

भ

A perfect mind comes from a perfect heart, not the heart known by a doctor's stethoscope but the heart which is the seat of God. It is claimed that realization of God in the heart makes it impossible for an impure or idle thought to cross the mind.

—"MAHATMA" M. K. GANDHI

THE HIGHEST HELP

भ

Spiritual knowledge is the only thing that can destroy our miseries forever; any other knowledge removes wants only for a time. It is only with the knowledge of the Spirit that the root cause of want is destroyed forever; so helping man spiritually is the highest help that can be given him.

—SWAMI VIVEKANANDA

2

THE QUEST

❧

The quest begins when we start asking the Big Questions: Who am I? Whence do I come? Whither do I go? What must I do? As Socrates observed, the unreflective life is not worth living. Yet, many people never pause long enough to ask Why am I alive? until they are thrown into a crisis. Perhaps a loved one dies or they themselves are facing a life-threatening disease. Then their awareness surfaces momentarily from the hubbub of daily life, and they can breathe the more rarefied air of metaphysical spaces.

The sages invite us to make self-reflection an integral part of our everyday living and not wait until disaster strikes. For then it could be too late to realign ourselves with the deeper purpose of human existence: to discover our true nature, which is the immortal Consciousness.

The quest is inherently paradoxical, for the great masters tell us that in our true nature we already are fully liberated and blessed with unalloyed happiness. But we do not know this, and even when we have encountered teachings that show us the truth about ourselves, we still do not experience our intrinsic freedom and bliss. To achieve liberation we must turn to consistent spiritual practice, for which there are no substitutes.

Because of this inbuilt paradox, the quest can be both exciting and frustrating. It can be exciting because there are desirable new vistas and possibilities, and it can be quite frustrating because the mind can see far ahead, but without the medium of steady discipline it cannot transport us to those new places.

The quest thus turns us into seekers. Since our contemporary culture offers us little spiritual guidance, our search will likely take us in all kinds of directions. Many of our explorations will dead-end, but even those apparent failures contribute to our inner growth, as long as we continue to keep our desire for self-knowledge alive.

In due course, we will discover a path that appeals to and makes sense to us. Then our quest becomes more focused, and instead of merely looking for we start finding ourselves. One day, this journey of self-discovery will flower into full-fledged Self-realization, the recovery of our true nature as pure, blissful, eternal Consciousness.

IN SEARCH OF LIGHT

❧

Man is a seeker. He dwells amid shadows and seeks for light.

—Sri Ananda Acharya

OVERCOMING LIMITATIONS

❧

All bondages are galling whether it is a bondage of the senses or the mind or the vital force. Any limitation torments and life appears to be like a noose being tightened round our necks. That is what is there at the bottom of man's restlessness.

—Vimala Thakar

DIGGING UP THE HIDDEN TREASURE

୬

Treasures lie in the womb of the earth, fire is latent in wood, and milk is in the udder of a cow. However, one has to take certain actions to acquire them. In the same way, even though the Supreme Principle is within us, a person who wishes to attain it must use the right means. This is necessary because we have been going in the wrong direction for such a long time. Even a person of discrimination and exalted vision must make some effort in order for that Principle to manifest for him completely.

—SWAMI MUKTANANDA

DISCOVERING MIRACLES WITHIN

୬

There are so many great treasures and miracles within you, so many magical possibilities hidden inside you. Through discipline, you can make them manifest for you, and in this way, you can make the earth a greater paradise.

—SWAMI CHIDVILASANANDA

LEARNING THE GREAT LESSON

~

The most important thing in life is neither marriage, nor a degree at a university, nor living in comfort and plenty. It is the will to learn. Unless we learn great lessons in life, we vegetate and fail to accomplish the purpose of life.

The region of consciousness is infinite; the sea of our mind is replete with priceless pearls. To live is to expand the horizon of our life and to discover the pearls of knowledge daily.

—HARI PRASAD SHASTRI

THE QUEST

~

The inner meaning of life does not readily reveal itself; it must be searched for. Such a search is the Quest.

When a man begins to seek out his real nature, to find the truth of his real being, he begins to follow the Quest.

The Quest is a veritable re-education of the self, leading in its turn to a noble transcendence of the self.

Some come to the truth in a roundabout way. The Quest is direct.

The Quest is spiritual mountaineering.

—PAUL BRUNTON

ASKING THE RIGHT QUESTIONS

ॐ

What is all this universe, this life, birth, death? What is the purpose of all this? What is at the bottom of all this? What is the goal of all these activities? Remain in these questions for as long as you can, remain longer and longer, you will know the Truth . . . which state is the natural desire of everybody in unclouded moments.

—SHIVAPURI BABA

LONGING FOR LIBERATION

ॐ

Your desire for realization is the strongest proof of your progress in the past and of your success in the future. Be sure that your longing for realization is greater than your love for life. Be not downhearted. The result may not seem proportionate to your efforts. The more you fail the nearer you are to the goal. Failure makes the soul more resolved to master success. . . . Direct the forces of the body towards the mind and the forces of the mind towards the soul.

—SRI ANANDA ACHARYA

THE BIG QUESTION

There is only one fundamental question: "Who am I?" Without knowing ourselves, nothing has any validity and our thought must breed illusion. In the inquiry into our real nature is the whole meaning of existence. All else is preliminary or superfluous.

—DAVID FRAWLEY

YEARNING TO GROW

Yearning is a part of the beginning of anybody's practice. You have to yearn to grow. You can't want it one day, but not the next, and expect to make any real progress. You have to begin with some steady, inner hunger.

—SWAMI CHETANANANDA

ASPIRING TO WISDOM'S LIGHT

❧

The deep yearning of the ego is for that which enables it to break the limitations and to stand tiptoe on the high hill to salute the rising sun of supreme wisdom.

—HARI PRASAD SHASTRI

3

THE TEACHER— GUIDING LIGHT

❧

Only the crazy or arrogant would set out to build or repair a computer without a manual or verbal instructions from a qualified technician. Likewise, in the absence of proper guidance, Yoga practice is also set on a course for failure. Such guidance may be found in various forms. It is possible to learn something about Yoga through books, audiotapes, videos, and CDs, but beyond the simplest of postures (*asana*), personal instruction is necessary.

There is, however, an important difference between a Yoga teacher (*acarya* or *upadhyaya* in the Sanskrit language) and a *guru*. Hopefully, a Yoga teacher is someone who is knowledgeable about the various philosophical ideas and practices of Yoga. He or she should also have attained a level of competence in the actual performance of the various yogic techniques. A *guru*, however, is not merely knowledgeable, but rather, by virtue of his or her self-mastery, functions primarily as a spiritual transmitter: He or she continuously radiates peace, love, and compassion. In his or her company, it is much easier to experience the same desirable qualities and also to reach higher states of consciousness.

The etymological meaning of the term *guru* is "he who is weighty," that is, he whose knowledge and wisdom count. According to a deeper explanation, the word's two syllables—*gu* and *ru*—respectively signify "darkness" and "destruction." Thus a *guru* is someone who dispels our spiritual darkness by putting us in touch with our true Self. Because our spiritual destiny is clearly more important than any possible knowledge we can acquire in the course of a lifetime, the *guru* also is far more important than any other kind of teacher.

Teachers have students, but *gurus* have disciples. This suggests a significant difference in relationship. Discipleship involves not only intellectual learning but inner growth based on a strong spiritual connection with a Yoga master. Therefore the disciple must be committed to self-transcendence, just as the *guru*'s only real interest is in making a master out of the disciple. Discipleship revolves around the pursuit of Self-realization, or enlightenment, and it is built on lifelong *discipline*. It is not surprising, therefore, that there are numerous Yoga students but few genuine disciples. While there are many benefits at the level of student—not least among them good health and fitness—the full power of Yoga manifests at the level of disciple.

In my book *Holy Madness*, I examined the *guru*-disciple relationship in some detail and also addressed the challenges and disappointments many Western students have experienced with their *gurus*. I am often asked how we can find the right teacher for us, and my answer is always the same: Prepare yourself! Examine a teacher carefully before making a commitment to him or her. A good teacher will do the same with you.

A HELPING HAND FROM HEAVEN

❧

Heaven lies within and without us, it is true. But in most cases, only by the intervention of some authentic spiritual genius do we seem able to translate this into actuality for ourselves.

No seeker is so wise, so informed, so perfect, or so balanced as not to need the constructive criticism and expert counsel of a true spiritual guide.

—PAUL BRUNTON

THE TEACHER IS AN INSTRUMENT

❧

The teacher helps you to become quiet and calm and to be free from your ego trip, and in that moment when you reach your Self, your natural energy flows out. The teacher is only an instrument to help you open your door. It would have opened of itself if you had been living naturally, but you don't have any faith in yourselves. You are always thinking, "Somebody must come and open my door," because you don't understand what you are.

—MUNISHREE CHITRABHANU

THE DUAL PURPOSE OF THE TEACHER

꒰ঌ

The role of the teacher is basically twofold: first, to arouse the deepest creative power of Life present within you; then, to support you as this power unfolds. As this happens, the creative power of Life makes you aware of the intimate inter-relationship of all spirit and matter, and of the oneness of all spirit. Supported by the teacher, you enter into an experience of union not only with the teacher, but also with that teacher in whom your own teacher is unified, and with the Teacher from whom all things have come forth. . . .

Furthermore, the physical teacher represents both a support and a resource—not a conspiracy to make you bound and dependent. The physical teacher doesn't exist to dominate your life, and no teacher with half a brain would even want to. What would be the point? Instead, the teacher is simply like a well from which you draw a clear, pure vitality which supports the process of your regeneration and transformation. It may take the form of advice, instruction, or a subtle but powerful exchange of energy; all of these are ways in which this funda-mental essence articulates its creative power.

—SWAMI CHETANANANDA

THE RIGHT APPROACH TO TEACHERS

༄

We ourselves create destructive illusions of leaders and follow-
ers, not only in the spiritual realm, but also in the political and
other realms as well. We cannot simply blame our leaders for
the illusions they may take upon themselves, once we have first
given our power over to them. We abuse our teachers when we
approach them, not with respect for truth, but with desire and
illusion, seeking recognition and reward. We abuse ourselves
when we project personality cults on people, rather than seeing them as they are. We are responsible for our reality, and it
is our own karma, or the effects of our actions, that we must
ultimately face, not the praise or blame we may receive from or
give to others. While this view appears harsh, in it alone is true
compassion, because it alone gives us the power to change our
destiny in a real way.

—DAVID FRAWLEY

TEACH YOURSELF

༄

No one is ever really taught by another; each of us has to
teach himself. The external teacher offers only the suggestion, which arouses the internal teacher, who helps us to understand things.

—SWAMI VIVEKANANDA

INNER *GURU*, OUTER *GURU*

ॐ

Many people have argued that a guru is not necessary, that the real guru is within us. This is true. But how many of us can claim to hear him, understand him, or follow his instructions?

Guru is the guiding light. He may be in the physical body, but his spirit soars high into realms unknown. It is our needs, not his, that bind him to the earth.

The inner guru is like the bombshell. . . . And the external guru is the detonator.

—SWAMI SATYASANGANANDA SARASWATI

4

FIRST STEPS ON THE PATH

॰ॐ॰

Beginnings are important, as they set the tone for what will follow. Thus beginners on the yogic path would do well to understand correctly what Yoga is all about and to then approach it accordingly. There is a humorous saying in Yoga circles that Yoga has been reduced to the practice of postures, and that postures have been reduced to stretching, and that stretching has been reduced to lengthening the hamstrings. Authentic Yoga is always a spiritual discipline, however, even when the focus is on the body, as it is in Hatha-Yoga.

Yoga aims at wholeness, and it can be fully appreciated only when we treat it as a whole. This means we must understand that it is a path to Self-realization—the recovery of our true nature, which is eternal, pure consciousness. Every single technique or practice of the highly diversified approach of Yoga has the same purpose: to set us free, to take us beyond the conditioning of our ego-personality, into the spacious realm of the Spirit, or higher Self (called *atman* or *purusha*).

As we set foot on the yogic path, we must right away

acknowledge that we have work to do on ourselves. This sense should stay with us until we are actually Self-realized, or liberated. All too often, sheer beginners fancy themselves as adepts and start assuming the role of teacher or even *guru*. Even when, after due preparation, we are called to teach others, we would be wise to remain learners—or, in traditional terms, to cultivate "beginner's mind." Otherwise we run the risk of self-delusion and isolation. We stop growing when we think there is nothing more to learn.

The best protection against going astray on the spiritual path is humility and integrity. That is why the yogic path begins not with the postures or meditation, as so widely believed, but with simple moral disciplines: nonharming, truthfulness, nonstealing, chastity, and greedlessness. After thirty-five years of attempting to practice Yoga as a spiritual discipline, I must confess that I am still struggling to perfect the first practice of the first limb of the eightfold path outlined by Sage Patanjali: nonharming (*ahimsa*). But when I look back on that stretch of time, I also can honestly say that I have grown spiritually in ways that I find encouraging. Thanks largely to my teachers, I have had many glimpses of Yoga's higher reaches, but I know that no ecstatic state (*samadhi*), however lofty, amounts to very much without firm grounding in the moral disciplines. For the ultimate goal of liberation depends on our psychological and moral integrity. The entire yogic process can be viewed as one of progressive self-purification. That is why there are no shortcuts to self-realization. We cannot trick our way there through drugs or other artifices. Our inner purity (or integrity) is the only doorway to freedom.

A COLORFUL PERSONALITY

ๆ

Take a clean and clear glass and throw on it a splash of yellow, or red, and blue, and again of yellow, pink or purple, and green. Such has become your personality over a lifetime of gathering experiences indiscriminately from the morning of childhood to the autumn of old age. Throughout life the only thing we do is paint our minds with such indiscriminate colors.

Personality is not Self. Personality is composite and an aggregate of many components. The Self is one, unalloyed. The personality is material, the Self is a spiritual energy. The personality changes constantly, the Self is unchanging. The personality is transient, the Self permanent. The Self is untouched, unaffected, ever pure, ever wise, ever free. It is neither attracted nor averse to anything and is never in ignorance because its very nature is consciousness. The personality is divided into many levels and planes, from the grossest to the finest, but the Self is indivisible.

—PANDIT USHARBUDH ARYA

BEYOND APPEARANCE

The whole point of spiritual work is to begin to understand that we are not what we appear to be. As we understand this more and more, we begin to find within ourselves a real and deep connection to the source of all Life.

—Swami Chetanananda

THE OTHER SIDE OF COMFORT

Those who want comfort in life have to seek conformity. The result is false compromise and hypocrisy, and the life without integrity becomes a patchwork.

—Swami Avyaktananda

THE TWO KEYS OF LIFE

The indestructible hall of human memory contains two keys. One is made of iron and is called Attachment, the other is made of gold and is called Detachment. The iron key opens the door of the house to lower life. The golden key opens the door of the house to higher life. Both the houses are in the unseen physiology of the human personality. At different periods of life, man wishes to open these doors, urged by inevitable impulse and interest, which shoot forth like meteoric showers from within the microcosmos.

—SRI ANANDA ACHARYA

THE TWELVE STEPS OF
SPIRITUAL RECOVERY

৯৮

1. We *admit* the fact that our conventional life is filled with suffering, because we do not know our true identity, the higher Self, which transcends space-time and body-mind. Instead we persist in the stubborn habit of assuming ourselves to be identical with a finite body-mind, thus creating the artificial center called the "ego." This amounts to a *denial* of the truth about human existence.

2. We begin to look and ask for *guidance* in our effort to cultivate a new outlook that embraces the reality of the higher Self and supersedes the artificial creation of an ego-personality. The means of doing so are varied—from a supportive spiritual environment to uplifting books.

3. We initiate *positive changes* in our behavior affirming that new outlook. It is not enough to read and talk about spiritual principles. Spirituality—Yoga—is a thoroughly practical affair.

4. We practice *self-understanding*, that is, we accept conscious responsibility for noticing our automatic programs and where they fall short of our new understanding of life.

5. We make a commitment to undergoing the *catharsis,* or purification, necessary to change our old cognitive and emotional patterns and stabilize the new outlook and disposition, replacing the egoic habit with the conscious practice of the presence of the higher Self.

6. We learn to be flexible and *open* to life so that we can continue to learn and grow on the basis of our new outlook.

7. We practice *humility* in the midst of our endeavors to mature spiritually. In this way we avoid the danger of psychic inflation.

8. We assume *responsibility* for what we have understood about life and the principles of spiritual recovery, applying our understanding to all our relationships so that we can be a benign influence in the world.

9. Guided by our new outlook, we work on the *integration* of our multiply divided psyche, allowing the higher Self to gradually replace the ego.

10. We cultivate real *self-discipline* in all matters, great and small.

11. We increasingly practice *spiritual communion,* which opens us to the higher Self, in which we are all connected. Through such communion and through continued growth in self-understanding, we become transparent to ourselves.

12. We open ourselves to the possibility of *bliss,* the breakthrough of the transcendental Reality into our consciousness, whereby the ego principle is unhinged and we fully recover our spiritual identity, the Self. Through this awakening, the world becomes transparent to us, and we are made whole.

—GEORG FEUERSTEIN

SHIFTING ONE'S OUTLOOK

❧

As our discrimination deepens and our detachment becomes stronger, our outlook and actions begin to change. Our clinging to the world is gradually lessened, and we awaken to the infinite human and spiritual potential that lies within us. This shift in outlook is an important step in our spiritual development, as it constitutes a turning from self-centeredness to God-centeredness, from selfishness to selflessness.

—SWAMI VIPRANANDA

KNOWING WHAT YOU DON'T WANT

❧

As we attempt to grow, the first things we learn are what we *don't* want. These are the easiest to recognize. Often, our initial experience shows us little more than this, but it is still a good thing. At least it reduces our confusion by one more degree and gives us some definite parameters within which to start to function.

—SWAMI CHETANANANDA

THE EIGHTFOLD PATH

෨

1. Avoid unrighteous behavior—*yama*.

2. Follow certain moral and spiritual precepts—*niyama*.

3. Learn to be still in body and mind, for where motion ceases, there begins the perception of God—*asana*.

4. While concentrating on the state of peace, practice control of the life force in the body—*pranayama*.

5. When your mind is your own, that is, under your control through *pranayama*, then you can give it to God—*pratyahara*.

6. Then begins meditation: first, concentrate on one of God's cosmic manifestations such as love, wisdom, joy—*dharana*.

7. What follows in meditation is an expansion of the realization of God's infinite omnipresent nature—*dhyana*.

8. When the soul merges as one with God, who is ever-existing, ever-conscious, ever-new Bliss, that is the goal—*samadhi*.

—PARAMAHANSA YOGANANDA

DON'T JUST SIT THERE

ॐ

All human beings want happiness, but they don't know how to go about it. They don't even know that there is work to be done and a discipline to be observed in order to obtain it. They think that just because they are here on earth they only need to eat, drink, sleep, earn a living and bring children into the world, and they should automatically be happy. But animals do pretty much the same things, so what is the difference? To be on earth is no guarantee of happiness. . . .

If you want happiness, don't just sit there and do nothing about it. You must go out and start looking for the elements that nourish it; and as these elements belong to the divine world, that is where you have to look for them. Once you find them you will love everyone and everything and be loved in return; you will understand things better, and you will have the power to create and achieve your aspirations.

—OMRAAM MIKHAËL AÏVANHOV

A SINGLE PURPOSE

The first thing necessary for Yoga is concentration of purpose. You have so many aims, so many purposes, that you are frittering away your little stock of energy in the attempt to accomplish them all. You are pursuing so many objects not because they are pleasant or profitable in themselves, but because you have neither found out the highest good of your life nor have you trained your will to realize it.

—SRI ANANDA ACHARYA

STOP NIBBLING

Those that only take a nibble here and a nibble there will never attain anything. . . . Those who really want to be yogis must give up, once for all, this nibbling at things. Take up one idea. Make that one idea your life—think of it, dream of it, live on that idea.

—SWAMI VIVEKANANDA

SINCERE EFFORT

❧

Divers search in the ocean for pearls; they don't find them every time. They may have to dive twenty or thirty times in the deep sea to get them—and even then they don't always succeed. Sometimes they may not find certain pearls for years, although the pearls are there. The diver is doing his duty, but he is not getting a reward. Each of us must likewise make repeated efforts in our own life. Always make an effort. But there should be sincerity in it.

—SWAMI RAMA

THE PRINCIPAL CONDITION
FOR SUCCESS

❧

The power needed in Yoga is the power to go through effort, difficulty or trouble without getting fatigued, depressed, discouraged or impatient and without breaking off the effort or giving up one's aim or resolution. A quiet vigilant but undistressed persistence is the best way to get the sadhana [yogic practice] done.

—SRI AUROBINDO

CONSISTENT CHEERFUL EFFORT

Practice demands an effort that is prolonged, stretching over a long duration. One cannot expect quick results on this path. There is nothing like instant Yoga. It requires a continuous effort spread over a number of years. Moreover this effort has to be uninterrupted. A spasmodic effort can never lead a person anywhere. To put in an effort for some time and then to retire in hibernation in order to rest on one's oars is of no use at all if one is really serious about journeying into the land of Yoga. But there is something more about this effort regarding which Patanjali speaks. . . . The effort must have a quality of cheerfulness about it. Yoga is not a Path of Woe; it is indeed a Way of Joy. If the effort is prolonged and uninterrupted and yet lacks this quality of joy then it is hardly of any worth at all. The effort must have an element of passion about it, for one cannot go to the door of Reality like a skeleton, completely squeezed out. The journey on the path requires great energy.

—ROHIT MEHTA

TRANSFORM YOUR MIND
THROUGH STUDY

❧

By this constant intake of spiritual ideas through daily study, gradually there comes about a process of mind-transformation. The old mind is gradually eliminated and a new mind is created within you, a new mind which always thinks spiritually, which always is in a state of awareness.

—SWAMI CHIDANANDA

SELF-OBSERVATION

❧

In order to make progress in any aspect of life, it is essential to develop your willpower and your personal strength. Often, however, when you decide to develop your willpower, you may resolve to do dramatic things, but this can actually cause problems for you, because if you cannot yet do what you resolve, then you will find that your strength and your willpower are being damaged rather than developed.

If you sincerely want to develop personal strength and willpower, you should first learn to keep yourself open and be an observer of yourself until you observe that your willpower has become dynamic. Instead of making such dramatic resolutions, simply make yourself open to observing yourself and decide to experiment in observing yourself.

—SWAMI RAMA

THE POISON OF FORCED DISCIPLINE

࿐

You cannot control the mind by forcible discipline; that is, by denying it all that is pleasurable. Discipline of the mind by force is like putting a snake in a covered basket. It will bite as soon as it gets an opportunity. However, if we remove its poison fangs, it becomes completely harmless. Similarly, the poison fangs of our mind, which are lust, anger, greed, attachment and pride or egoism, can be removed only by spiritual practice.

—MAHARAJ CHARAN SINGH

UPLIFT YOURSELF BY THE SELF

࿐

One should raise oneself by the Self.
One should not degrade oneself.
For the Self alone is the friend of the self,
and the self alone is the enemy of the Self.

—BHAGAVAD-GITA

5

CHALLENGING
THE EGO

࿐

According to the overwhelming testimony of Yoga masters and adepts of other spiritual traditions, in our true nature we are absolutely and eternally free, wide awake, and unsurpassably blissful. But this is not our day-to-day experience. Instead we find ourselves lodged in a particular body-mind from which we look out onto a world populated by countless others.

This sense of being located, even locked into, a particular body-mind is what Yoga calls the principle of individuation, or "I-maker" (*ahamkara*). The ego is a false identity by means of which we navigate through—or masquerade in—the familiar world of multiple subjects and objects. Often I am asked why, if our true nature comprises everything and everyone as an irreducible Singularity, we experience ourselves as insulated in a particular body-mind that is surrounded by countless others. There is no really satisfying answer to this conundrum. It is a simple fact. We are cultivating this false identity right now. We are not realizing who we really are—the One that transcends space and time and sustains the universe in its entirety. All our suffering stems from this ongoing error. To use religious language, no one has cast us out of paradise; rather we ourselves are preventing our entry into it.

Yoga is designed to help us remember who we are in truth—the singular Self (*atman* or *purusha*). Thus every single yogic practice seeks to undermine the ego illusion, our ongoing action of self-encapsulation. If it does not, it is not really Yoga.

Of course, dismantling our false self-sense is demanding emotionally. For our ego-identity is not merely a cognitive error that could be corrected easily by adopting the right view. Instead it comes with a good many emotional factors that can be grouped into two broad categories: likes and dislikes. Master Patanjali, the compiler of the well-known *Yoga-Sutra,* speaks of *raga* ("passionate attachment") and *dvesha* ("passionate recoil") as the engine that powers conventional life. They are our on-and-off switch. We are attached to pleasurable experiences, and avoid unpleasant ones. Whatever flavor our experiences may have, they all have the ego as their pivot and are feeding it.

We can learn to transcend the ego, gradually, by placing ourselves more and more in the position of the transcendental Self, which knows no likes and dislikes but simply witnesses all experiences and states of existence. As our capacity for witnessing—mindfulness—increases, we automatically slip more and more into our true nature. The way from self to Self—or from the ego to the ultimate I AM—demands courage, determination, and commitment, that is, continuous daily practice of self-transcendence in the innumerable circumstances that life presents to us.

THE TRUTH ABOUT US

❧

All our violence, all our competitiveness, all our terrific anxiety to survive is because we did not know from the beginning that we were IT.

—ALAN WATTS

IMPRISONED BY THE EGO

❧

We sit in the ego with all its limitations as in a prison and we do not know that we are prisoners, for we identify ourselves with it and blind ourselves by those very limitations. It is there and it has to be there, but it need not be there to imprison us or to narrow our outlook. The ego imprisons us, for instance, with its memories which keep us steeped in the past when the wisdom of the spirit is to live in the eternal now—which is all we have in reality and which alone is real for neither past nor future possess any reality.

—PAUL BRUNTON

THE EGO IS NOT AN ENTITY

࿇

The ego is not an entity but an activity. It is contraction of the field of Radiance.

—BUBBA FREE JOHN (ADI DA)

THE EGO AS CONTRACTION

࿇

God is the vast Self-awareness, or consciousness, that is the subtle essence of all things. The whole universe is an expression of the vitality of this consciousness, a subtle pulsation that interacts with itself. Through various stages of increasing contraction and density, this pure, undifferentiated awareness expresses itself as individual conscious events. It is here that the sense of "I" begins. Each "I," like a spiral current in the energy of Life, becomes conscious of itself, or self-aware. It comes to perceive itself as separate and distinct from the surrounding atmosphere and becomes aware of other "I's" around it. Here begins our sense of ego.

—SWAMI CHETANANANDA

THE ONLY FOE

We have to make a single community of this whole world. If there is anything that is to be treated as an alien, it is "me and mine." This "me and mine" is the worst enemy. This great enemy has to be killed, extirpated. Then only will this whole world become your own—of God—and full of peace and happiness.

—SWAMI PREMANANDA

WILLPOWER OVER EGO POWER

The power of ego is like a little pool. In that pool, an egotistical person lives like a frog—his world is small, his borders insecure, and from his perspective, only his own thoughts, feelings, and voice seem to be meaningful. But the power of will springs from the inner Self, from pure Being. It infuses the mind and body with enthusiasm, courage, an ever-growing curiosity to know, and the energy to act.

—PANDIT RAJMANI TIGUNAIT

THE ULTIMATE SHAPE-SHIFTER

❧

Ego can take many different forms and shapes. It is like the hydra. You cut off one head and another head replaces it. You cut off that head and you see a third head and a fourth head, ad infinitum. This is because in the manifest dimension, ego identity is the root of life, and if that ego identity is lost, then life as we know it no longer exists. It exists as light; life becomes light.

—SWAMI NIRANJANANANDA SARASWATI

THE EGO IS A HABIT

❧

The ego is nothing but memory, a set of definitions which are limiting. You strongly believe in these patterns you have yourself brought about and you mechanically repeat them. It is only habit that maintains them, makes them seem permanent. Let them go once and for all.

—JEAN KLEIN

WHITTLING AWAY THE EGO

⁊

One must gradually whittle away the ego, as though one is chipping at a piece of stone till the stone no longer exists—bit by bit. This . . . can take place only when there is exquisite awareness of one's day-to-day and moment-to-moment existence.

—SWAMI GITANANDA GIRI

SELF-CONTROL

⁊

One should control the self,
which is indeed difficult to control.
By controlling the self,
one gains happiness
now and in the future.

—*UTTARADHYAYANA-SUTRA*

6

THE GOOD LIFE

✦

We think of "the good life" as a life filled with comfort and pleasure, as our having a good time. In yogic terms, however, the good life is one dedicated to that which is good or virtuous, which is in some sense the opposite meaning. To our contemporary ears, *virtue* has a fuddy-duddy ring to it. In its Latin root, however, the word means not only moral merit but also valor, intrinsic quality, and power.

According to the *Shila-Samyukta-Sutra,* a Buddhist Yoga scripture, just as a legless person cannot walk, so an individual lacking in morality cannot become liberated. A morally sound life places us in a position of strength, for it mobilizes the spiritual resources that allow us to engage life more sanely and effectively, in consonance with the highest aspects of Nature: beauty and harmony.

Most Western practitioners *do* Yoga once or twice a week, by which they mean practicing the postures, deep breathing, or perhaps a little bit of meditation. Often the rest of their day is given over to the conventional mind, without resort to Yoga. The good life of Yoga, however, must be *lived* twenty-four hours per day. This includes work, interaction with others, sleep, eating, and sex. The *yogi* or *yogini* is expected to bring the witnessing consciousness, or mindfulness, to all these aspects of life, and Yoga offers many excellent guidelines for doing so.

The key in all things is balance. In fact, according to the *Bhagavad-Gita*, a Yoga classic, one of the definitions of Yoga is "evenness" (*samatva*). We must bring harmony to whatever we do, say, and think, and harmony is a manifestation of the principle of lucidity. All the myriad beings and things in Nature are composites of three principles or qualities (*guna*): the principle of lucidity (*sattva*), the principle of dynamism (*rajas*), and the principle of inertia (*tamas*). At the ordinary level of experience, they might manifest as daylight, dusk/dawn, and night; waking, dream, and deep sleep; wisdom, knowledge, and ignorance; kindness, meanness, and indifference; space, air, and solid ground; fresh organic fruit, cooked vegetables, and processed food; and so on.

The objective of Yoga, first and foremost, is to increase *sattva* in our body and mind—a process I call *sattvification*. Then when *sattva* predominates within us, that is, when our mind has reached a level of great lucidity, we can glimpse our true nature—the eternal witness. Then the switch from ego-identity to Self-Identity occurs, which establishes us in freedom and bliss. The cultivation of *sattva* calls for discipline relative to the body, the mind, and speech. One of the meanings of the Sanskrit word *yoga* is, in fact, "discipline."

THE MAGIC OF VIRTUE

> ৯

Spiritual virtues have a special magic about them: when you develop them within your personality, similar qualities proceed from others and are directed towards you. If you are compassionate towards others, compassion from an external source comes to you in a time of need.

—SWAMI JYOTIRMAYANANDA

SPIRITUAL LIFE AND MORALS

> ৯

Human life being an undivided whole, no line can ever be drawn between its different compartments, nor between ethics and politics. A trader who earns his wealth by deception only succeeds in deceiving himself when he thinks that his sins can be washed away by spending some amount of his ill-gotten gains on the so-called religious purposes. One's everyday life is never capable of being separated from one's spiritual being. Both act and react upon one another.

—"MAHAṬMA" M. K. GANDHI

SPIRITUAL RECIPROCITY

❧

If you want the surroundings to be of best use to you, be of best use to your surroundings. If you want your house to give you joy and comfort, be joyful in it, bring to it beautiful things. If you project love to the plants in your garden, they will reward you with beautiful flowers to give you joy. If you cultivate within yourself a natural state of kindness, compassion, love, and forgiveness, you will receive a thousandfold reward from the surroundings.

—MAHARISHI MAHESH YOGI

THE JOY OF SERVICE

❧

Compassionate service helps to alleviate the pain of those who are suffering. But its greater value lies in purifying the minds and hearts of those who render it. The satisfaction and joy you derive from rendering selfless service to someone in need is immense and everlasting. However, there is one danger—feeding your ego by identifying yourself as a generous, compassionate person. This is destructive both to you and to those to whom you render service.

—PANDIT RAJMANI TIGUNAIT

JOYOUS ACTION

❧

Duty and pity fall short of true compassion. Joy is present only when an act is born of wisdom, love, compassion and equanimity. Such action is joyful because it is not restrained by attachment nor burdened with worries and anxieties.

—THYNN THYNN

THE YOGA OF SELF-TRANSCENDING ACTION

❧

To action alone are you entitled, never to its fruit.
Let not the fruit of action be your motive.
Neither let there be any attachment to inaction.

Abiding in Yoga, do your work without attachment
and with being balanced in success or failure.
Balance is called Yoga.

—*BHAGAVAD-GITA*

EGO-TRANSCENDING ACTION

᠍

When acting and actor disappear,
All actions become correct.

—MILAREPA

COMPETING *WITH* OTHERS

᠍

When we compete without thinking to "win," valuing everyone's efforts equally, competition can be a very positive
motivating force. It can teach us to appreciate our abilities
more deeply, and it can lead to an appreciation and a greater
respect for the capabilities of others as well. Unfortunately,
because competition is the road to success and power in
business, politics, and education, even in social interactions,
it is usually used to gain selfish aims. Instead of competing
with others, we compete *against* them. When competition becomes combat, it loses its power to inspire, and becomes instead a form of pressure which creates disharmony in our
minds and senses, upsetting the natural balance of our lives.

—TARTHANG TULKU

WORK AND WORSHIP

ॐ

Work and worship must go hand in hand. It is very good if one can devote oneself solely to spiritual practices. But how many can do that? Two types of men can sit still without work. One is the idiot, who is too dull to be active. The other is the saint who has gone beyond all activity. Work is a means to the state of meditation. Instead of working for yourself, work for the Lord. Know that you are worshipping the Lord through your work.

—SWAMI BRAHMANANDA

FLOWER POWER

ॐ

No self-centered attitude, no self-immolation, no violence against ourselves, all these things belong to the past and it is an old-fashioned way of behaving. Why not be like the flowers in the field without any reason? They live, they blossom, they expand. Their perfume is swept in the air by the wind and it is not contaminated by ideas, duties, motivations. Those things would twist the flowers in different directions.

—SWAMI KARMANANDA SARASWATI

CHOOSE YOUR FRIENDS WISELY

ॐ

It is the wisest wisdom to select only those as friends who will help towards the blossoming of the Tree of Divinity within you. The character, tastes and opinions of your friend are constantly undergoing change, for the better or for the worse. You must carefully watch the shifting color of his ideal and decide whether his company is dragging you down or pulling you up. Remember that introspection is the only lever of conduct. Question your soul more often than you consult your watch or your barometer.

In true friendship, mutual love produces a constant upward movement of the two souls. . . . There is nothing in the world too precious to give to win a friend with whom you may tramp together round the universe of the sun and the universe of the soul.

—SRI ANANDA ACHARYA

TRUTH REIGNS SUPREME

ॐ

There is nothing higher than Truth.
There is no sin greater than falsehood.
Therefore, with one's whole being,
one should seek refuge in Truth.

—*MAHANIRVANA-TANTRA*

UNTRUTH UNDERMINES ALL

❧

Untruth is the breeding ground of all sin. There is nothing more unclean than untruth. Untruth has a wonderful capacity to vitiate all your life. Before you know it untruth brings you face to face with fear. Untruth is very proficient in giving rise to endless complexes, evils and diseases without your ever knowing anything about its processes. Untruth lands you in folly, fear, hypocrisy and false pride. Anyone who gives quarter to untruth even once will find that all sorts of impurities will enter into him by the backdoor. So the foundation stone of the spiritual endeavour is purity of life and purity means truthful behavior.

—VIMALA THAKAR

HUMILITY AND GRATITUDE

❧

Humility and gratitude go hand in hand. The feeling of gratitude is an interaction between the mind and the body. Both will benefit from it. Awareness increases so that we become grateful for everything we are given. We have to learn, literally learn, to be grateful for what we receive day by day, simply to balance the criticism that, day by day, we voice because of powerful emotions.

—SWAMI SIVANANDA RADHA

HUMILITY THROUGH
SELF-UNDERSTANDING

Humility is an experience of the commonality of all human beings. It leads to a balanced outlook on human nature that takes into account all the strengths and failings each of us is subject to. To be truly humble requires taking an honest look at ourselves, and coming to clearly know our abilities and weaknesses. When our personal evaluation is honest, we can respect who we are, and this deep acceptance of our nature leads to a wider understanding and greater respect for others. We are motivated to help others with their problems and to support them in cultivating their capabilities. We see that we all share similar goals of happiness and fulfillment; we are all subject to similar problems and difficulties.

—TARTHANG TULKU

PATIENCE

Why do we hear so little about patience today? There almost seems a conspiracy in our modern civilization to counsel just the opposite: be impatient, be angry, "look out for number one." But what is life without patience? . . . We seldom realize what power there is in patience. All the energy consumed in exploding against others, in retaliating, in unkind words, in the anger that brings grief to others and ulcers to ourselves—all that energy can be harnessed as positive, creative power, simply by learning patience. . . . Imagine someone who cannot be disturbed even if you are rude or unkind to him. Imagine someone who moves closer to you when you get angry, instead of running away; someone who keeps showing respect even when you try to strike out and hurt him. Simply being around such people is a joy. Their patience rubs off. Gradually we want to be like them. When we have a selfish impulse, we reject it; we have seen something higher. Once we have an ideal like this to live up to, we try to stretch ourselves a little every day; we see opportunities in every challenge.

—EKNATH EASWARAN

SICKENING SPEED

❧

A mind that is fast is sick.
A mind that is slow is sound.
A mind that is still is divine.

—MEHER BABA

LUMINOUS SLEEP

❧

Before going to sleep, fill your mind and heart with a
thought, and inspiration, a luminous image, and you will
wake up in the morning purified and regenerated.

—OMRAAM MIKHAËL AÏVANHOV

NOCTURNAL YOGI

❧

The rejuvenating effects of sleep are due to man's temporary unawareness of body and breathing. The sleeping man becomes a yogi; each night he unconsciously performs the yogic rite of releasing himself from bodily identification, and of merging the life force with healing currents in the main brain region and in the six subdynamos [the *cakras*] of his spinal centers. Unknowingly, the sleeper is thus recharged by the cosmic energy that sustains all life.

—PARAMAHANSA YOGANANDA

7

TAMING THE
EMOTIONS

୬

All spirituality, Yoga included, has self-understanding, self-discipline, and self-transcendence at its core. A good part of the work confronting *yogis* and *yoginis* concerns the realm of the emotions.

While we are embodied, our true nature, which is pure Consciousness, is obscured by countless thoughts and emotions, many of them of the afflicted variety. We constantly become involved in them as if *they* were our true nature. When anger, fear, or jealousy arises, we say, "I am angry," "I am afraid," or "I am jealous." In each case we do not merely witness the emotion but identify with it. Then, in that state of emotional identification—which is really a misidentification, since we are the transcendental Self—we take particular actions. Again we identify with the notion of being an agent who initiates limited activities. Those actions have repercussions, which then lead to renewed mental and emotional states with which we identify. In this way, we keep the illusion of being a particular ego-personality (or body-mind) going indefinitely, reaping both pleasure and pain.

As Yoga practitioners, we are called to not be attached to particular states of mind and especially to go beyond their negative manifestations—such as anger, fear, lust, hatred, envy, jealousy, or greed. "Going beyond" does not mean repressing them, but placing ourselves in our core Identity, the transcendental Self, by becoming the witness of our manifold activities. As the witness, we get in touch with our innate bliss, which then outshines all other possible emotions and thoughts. Witnessing brings clarity and simplicity into our mind and life.

We don't have to struggle with negative emotions; rather through our witnessing they gradually defuse themselves, giving us more and more inner space, or tranquillity. It is in that peaceful space that the work of Yoga can flourish. One of the great masters of medieval Christian spirituality, Meister Eckhart, observed in one of his sermons that we can offer God nothing better than peace. For it is then that the Divine can effect the miracle of transformation in us. Meister Eckhart represents the zenith of Christian spirituality, and his teachings show remarkable parallels to the highest expressions of yogic wisdom.

The more we activate the principle of *sattva*—lucidity—in ourselves, the more our mind becomes a still, calm pool. Ordinarily, its surface is broken by countless ripples, which blur our vision and reflect back to us the fragmented self (the ego-personality) rather than the whole Self, our true nature. According to Master Patanjali, we must control the fluctuations of the mind if we desire to catch sight of the transcendental Self. Control (*nirodha*) is an important concept of Yoga. It goes hand in hand with the concept of cultivating an introspective mind (*pratyak-cetana*), which alone is the antidote to our normal scattered state of consciousness.

Every action—even a mere thought or emotion—provokes a

corresponding reaction. This is the mechanism behind what the adepts of Yoga call *karma*. Bad karma is action/reaction that keeps us bound to the state of unenlightenment, with all its consequences. Good karma is action/reaction that promotes those qualities that are conducive to harmony, peace, happiness, and ultimately enlightenment.

Yoga helps us dive deep into our unconscious, where the karmic seeds for our egoic thoughts and behavior are found. On the way into the hidden recesses of our mind, we encounter all sorts of emotions that require cleaning out or transmutation. All the practices of Yoga are geared toward accomplishing this housecleaning and setting us free.

FOLLOW YOUR HEART

❧

Without heart, everything else counts for nought. Unless the heart expands, nothing else will avail.

—Swami Akhandananda

FEELINGS AND DESTINY

❧

Your feelings are creating your fortune every moment of the day and night. If you are not sufficiently wary, they will create a world of misfortune for you. A wish is like a mold and the flux of events is like molten metal. Choose a good mold and the shape of your life will be good.

—Sri Ananda Acharya

EMOTIONAL PURIFICATION

❧

If you have not purified your emotions, the lightning rod of spirituality will only shock you rather than illuminate you.

—Pandit Usharbudh Arya

TAMED EMOTIONS

Emotions in themselves are not bad, but when running wild they can be extremely damaging. Even love, when not shared, not given freely and generously, becomes self-love which turns destructively back on the individual. When emotions are directed, they are a source of strength for great achievements. Through the power of emotions men and women have overcome their limitations and attained a higher purpose in life. Emotions channeled through a Mantra towards the Divine can take you close to God.

—SWAMI SIVANANDA RADHA

LIBERATING EMOTION

❧

The best response to negative emotion is to allow it to self-liberate by remaining in nondual awareness, free of grasping and aversion. If we can do this, the emotion passes through us like a bird flying through space; no trace of its passage remains. The emotion arises and then spontaneously dissolves into emptiness.

In this case, the karmic seed is manifesting—as emotion or thought or bodily sensation or an impulse toward particular behaviors—but because we do not respond with grasping or aversion, no seed of future karma is generated. Every time that envy, for example, is allowed to arise and dissolve in awareness without our becoming caught by it or trying to repress it, the strength of the karmic tendency toward envy weakens. There is no new action to reinforce it. Liberating emotion in this way cuts karma at its root. It is as if we burn the karmic seeds before they have an opportunity to grow into trouble in our life.

—TENZIN WANGYAL RINPOCHE

EMOTIONAL CHAIN REACTION

⫘

He who understands anger understands pride; he who understands pride understands conceit; he who understands conceit understands greed; he who understands greed understands attachment; he who understands attachment understands aversion; he who understands aversion understands delusion; he who understands delusion understands conception; he who understands conception understands birth; he who understands birth understands death; he who understands death understands hell; he who understands hell understands animal existence; he who understands animal existence understands pain.

Therefore the sage should avoid anger, pride, conceit, greed, attachment, aversion, delusion, conception, birth, death, hell, animal existence, and pain.

—VARDHAMANA MAHAVIRA

ENSNARED CONSCIOUSNESS

⫘

A consciousness suffused with the taints
of likes and dislikes is unable to soar,
like a bird caught in a snare.

—YOGA-VASISHTHA

JOY BEYOND FUN

৵

I don't think any sensitive person can be satisfied with having fun, no matter how much of it we may cram into our lives. Our need is not for pleasure but for joy—a deep sense of fulfillment that not only never leaves us but actually increases with the passage of time. Fun is living for ourselves; joy comes from living for others, giving our time and love to a purpose greater than ourselves.

—EKNATH EASWARAN

MIND'S WEB

৵

There is no fire like passion.
There is no grasping like ill will.
There is no snare like delusion.
There is no river like craving.

—*DHAMMAPADA*

ADAMANTINE DESIRE

～

Chemically speaking, diamonds and coal are both nothing but carbon, but there is a big difference between the two. Desire for the world is like coal. Desire for God-realization is like a diamond. Worldly desire can be transformed into spiritual aspiration—just as mere coal is transformed into diamonds—when a constant effort is directed to control *kama* [desire] and to redirect it in a proper way.

—SWAMI JYOTIRMAYANANDA

THE TRUTH ABOUT DESIRE

～

Desire is necessary to human life and the spiritual desires do not extinguish desire, but only give it another and higher direction. If there were no desire there could be no universe, for God could not make this universe if He did not desire to do so.

—PAUL BRUNTON

FACING THE TIGER

༄

I was sitting in meditation in the forests of Arbudachal. Something was moving nearby. I opened my eyes. It was the king of the forests himself standing at a distance of less than ten feet—a big, beautiful body, nine feet long. What splendour he carried about him! What a shapely form, what colour, what eyes, what majesty of bearing. I was lost in admiration. Fear had simply no room to come in between us. The delight of feeling for beauty conquers fear.

I continued to be lost in admiration. We exchanged glances. The king of the forest must have been wondering who it was who was sitting so blissfully in his own domains. It was only a brief encounter, just for a few seconds during which I could feel the warmth and the smell of his body. And then he stepped away. On his way back he turned his face, looked at me and proceeded further. There was no reason for him to behave in any other manner. If there were any vibrations of fear within me at the moment, if I had even perspired out of fear, the very smell of the perspiration would have induced him to attack me.

—VIMALA THAKAR

CONQUERING FEAR

❧

Fear of fear is far worse than fear itself. Most fear vanishes when the fear of fear is destroyed. . . .

A steady mind is the most effective antidote to fear. Do not let fear terrorize you, for fearful situations create mental unsteadiness. Learn the lesson of the dove in the story I will now relate to you.

Doves are extremely afraid of cats. Once a dove spied a cat walking some distance away. Even though the cat was far away, the dove crouched down trembling, closed his eyes, and clung frozenly to his perch. By closing his eyes to shut out the sight of the cat, the dove believed he could chase fear away and keep the cat from seeing him. Impossible! By blinding himself with fear, doesn't the foolish dove merely make himself easy prey for the cat?

—Swami Shri Kripalvanandji

HARNESSING THE ENERGY OF ANGER

❧

By expressing anger to another person, you harm yourself in two ways. First, you block channels of communication with the other person, which, for better or worse, are part of the flow-pattern that nourishes your life—even if that person represents an endless source of frustration for you. Secondly, you contract your understanding of the particular moment. The energy which you express as anger should be more appropriately used to expand this understanding.

If you refrain from expressing your anger, then it becomes possible for three things to happen. First of all, you have the opportunity to recognize the senselessness of anger, and the need to do something progressive. Next, you become aware of your responsibility for the difficulty, whatever it may be. This allows you to begin to turn it around inside for a while, after which you can articulate it not as frustration, but as a higher understanding. Finally, in doing this, you can change whatever it is that you've been doing to generate such situations. You can also, at the same time, free the other person from what maybe has been unconscious behavior, developed in reaction to you or to some misunderstanding between you.

Anger is really only a demonstration of some blockage in your own system, and not in anybody else's.

—Swami Chetanananda

MELTING AWAY ANGER

❧

Once you begin to watch your anger, you will make an interesting discovery. You will find that as soon as you know you are angry, your anger will melt away by itself. It is very important that you watch without likes or dislikes. The more you are able to look at your own anger without making judgments, without being critical, the more easily the anger will dissipate.

—THYNN THYNN

OVERCOMING NEGATIVITY
THROUGH WITNESSING

❧

The harder we struggle against our negativity, the more energy we give it and the stronger it becomes. The only way out is to watch. If you are maintaining your stance as a witness, you will catch your mind spinning out a string of negative comments. Then, you can intervene.

—ARUNA BHARGAVA

THE PURSUIT OF POWER

༄

The pursuit of power derives from the separate self. As a separate self we must pursue power because as a separate self we are nothing, a mere point of weakness and alienation. Power does not dissolve this sense of separation but only gives it a false strength.

—DAVID FRAWLEY

OVERCOMING ANGER

༄

The method to diminish our afflictions is meditation. For example, if anger is our main problem, we need to engage in doing specific meditations that develop compassion and love. When we are angry we have the wish to harm, to beat, to hit, to insult. As a remedy we need to develop compassion and love, the main causes of our mental peace and relaxation.

Compassion is the attitude wishing that all sentient beings could be free from suffering. We meditate in order to make this attitude manifest, to transform our mind into the nature of compassion. Having accomplished this, we try to hold this attitude in our mind and focus upon it. However, it will probably quickly disappear and we will find that we need to make an effort to develop it once again. At first the compassion we generate will last only a minute, or maybe just a second, but by developing it again and again it will come to last for five minutes, ten minutes, fifteen minutes, and so on, gradually becoming more and more stable. By making a constant effort day after day, some result will definitely come—the hatred and anger will lessen and we will gradually find ourselves becoming more patient and relaxed.

We can also meditate on love to overcome anger. In this context, love does not refer to the kind of love we mean when we say, "I love you." Generally, when we say, "I love you," we mean, "I am attached to you." Real love is the mental attitude wishing that all sentient beings have happiness. Through meditation we make this kind of mind manifest, we transform our mind into the nature of love and then hold and focus on this attitude. This is what is known as meditation on love.

—GESHE JAMPA GYATSO

AMBITION

What are you looking for in life? Are you a race horse that can beat every other horse to the finish line? Or are you on your way to becoming a meditative saint? Most people lead the lives of race horses, wanting to beat every neighbor to the finish line, whatever that finish line may be.

—PANDIT USHARBUDH ARYA

OVERCOMING JEALOUSY

❦

To overcome jealousy, try to adopt a more advanced philo-sophical perspective. Begin to see yourself as a cosmic being, not as an individual, and all personalities as manifestations of the same Self.

Learn to see every human being as you would see your child or another near and dear relative. As such, they are all deserving of great joy. The happiness of all beings is yours. The world is your family, your own limb, your own Self. In the vast treasury of bliss that your inner Self enjoys, there is an abundance for all, and more is eternally forthcoming.

—SWAMI JYOTIRMAYANANDA

CRITICISM IS ALWAYS CONSTRUCTIVE

❦

No one teaches us in school how to cope with criticism, turn-ing it to our advantage.... To rectify this, we offer here the world's shortest course on "Censure Management." Never cringe before criticism. Take it like a man, even if you're a woman. Winnow the true from the false, then keep both. Smile at it. Better yet, understand it; best of all, learn from it. And never, never offer offenders quid pro quo. End of course.

—SATGURU SIVAYA SUBRAMANIYASWAMI

CORRECT FAULT-FINDING

Be like an eye always seeing your own faults,
But be like a blind person toward the faults of others.
—ATISHA

DON'T JUDGE OTHERS

Let us guard against judging others. The yogic attitude is to mind our own actions and not to be self-styled detectives of God. When we act, one hundredth part of our personality is expressed outwardly and ninety-nine parts are expressed entirely on other levels. So to take one detail and judge the whole personality of man from that standpoint is surely wrong. The human personality is not merely a machine that acts. A sewing machine is judged on how it sews, but man is not a machine. He has deep complexes hidden in his personality, sometimes not known to himself.
—HARI PRASAD SHASTRI

HEALING WORDS

Learn to speak gently and lovingly, not only to human beings but also to animals, flowers, birds, trees and the whole
of nature, for this is a divine habit. He who knows how to ut-
ter words that inspire and vivify possesses a magic wand in
his mouth, and his words will never be spoken in vain. . . .

—OMRAAM MIKHAËL AÏVANHOV

PEACE OVERCOMES ENMITY

The principal source of happiness is inner peace. Someone
who has already had practice in developing this peace, who
already has a certain experience of it, will not be easily trou-
bled by ordinary enemies. However, hatred, malice, and spite
will immediately destroy this mental calmness. The true enemy, therefore, is malice. External enemies may be real enemies for a certain time, but it is quite conceivable that one
day instead of harming us they may turn into friends. But
the inner enemy will always be our enemy—in the beginning,
midway through, and at the end; it is impossible that it will
ever become useful to us.

—THE DALAI LAMA

THE FRUIT OF NONVIOLENCE

❧

Nonviolence creates an ability in you to recognize the underlying unity of life. You then can gain great comfort in realizing that you are not separate or alone, but instead, part of the magnificent system of the world's life. You do not, then, feel threatened by any life form, because any life form would be observed as part of yourself. All life would be your life, supported by the spiritual body.

—ALICE CHRISTENSEN

GENTLENESS

❧

Learn to be gentle with others and learn to be gentle with yourself. Violent people are violent because they are not at peace with themselves. So be gentle to yourself. Then you will be able to express gentleness in your mind, action, and speech. It will come spontaneously.

—SWAMI RAMA

CHEERFULNESS

❧

Cheerfulness is a spontaneous expression of a purified heart and a steady mind. A clear mind is naturally blessed with cheerfulness, and a cheerful person spontaneously loves all and hates none. A cheerful person is fulfilled within, and this cheerfulness overflows, affecting everyone who comes near. On the other hand, an impure mind teems with countless conflicts. Spiritually speaking, a person with such a mind is empty. One who is empty envies those who are fulfilled, and easily becomes angry and vengeful. Therefore, it is of utmost importance to cultivate those divine qualities that purify the heart and steady the mind, thereby allowing cheerfulness to unfold spontaneously.

—PANDIT RAJMANI TIGUNAIT

PILGRIMAGE TO COMPASSION

❧

Since all living beings—animals, birds, insects, and human beings—are worthy of compassion, the realm of compassion is very vast. The pilgrimage to the domain of compassion is an auspicious one, because compassion also embraces strangers—not just those close to us.

—SWAMI SHRI KRIPALVANANDJI

INFINITE COMPASSION

For as long as space endures
and the world exists,
may my own existence bring about
the end of all suffering in the world.

—SHANTIDEVA

HAPPINESS FOR EVERYONE

As we are all human beings living on earth among countless
other human beings, our happiness is intimately connected
to that of others. It is hard to imagine personal happiness
detached or separate from the happiness of others. For it is
certain that if we aspire to happiness, we must be deeply concerned about the happiness of all humankind.

—THE DALAI LAMA

8

MASTERING THE
MATERIAL WORLD

જી

We are so embroiled in the needs and wants of the physical body and its survival that we tend to consider the material world to be "all there is." This unfortunate, impoverished view of life leads to the erroneous assumption that when the body drops off, we are altogether annihilated. In the meantime, we anxiously cling to matter as if it were our salvation.

We work frantically to achieve material security and comfort, sometimes at the expense of our health and sanity. Accumulating wealth is difficult and often filled with anxiety. Safeguarding it once we have acquired it also has its problems and attendant fears. When wealth diminishes, panic is engendered, followed by a renewed struggle to regain lost ground. We are attached to material things by numerous emotional cords that get yanked whenever material loss occurs. We sometimes even collapse emotionally and give up on life.

It is better to focus on nonattachment and the other great virtues of Yoga, which create inner plenty, contentment, and the sense that we are being taken care of. When we feel inwardly rich, our material circumstance cannot fill us with anxiety or tension. We simply do what is appropriate and trust that life—or the Divine—will meet our needs. Sometimes people ask me: "What if our needs are not met?" First of all, we must distinguish between needs and wants, and often what we have come to regard as needs are, on closer inspection, merely wants. Moreover, there is a sense among Yoga adepts that when we truly engage the spiritual process, we are given support from the subtle (spiritual) dimension. We may not own a villa or even a car—spiritual practitioners, in fact, are seldom blessed with material riches—but we also will not lack the necessary means for continuing on the path.

We can only master the material world when we have succeeded in self-mastery.

TRUE WEALTH

✌

This spiritual work is your only wealth, the only thing that can truly be said to belong to you. All the rest can be taken from you; only your work will be yours forever.

—OMRAAM MIKHAËL AÏVANHOV

RENUNCIATION BEYOND CONTROL

✌

It is necessary that we renounce everything. Yet the nature of this renunciation has usually been misunderstood and its sense of freedom lost. Renunciation does not mean giving up something, like giving up material things in order to gain something spiritual. Renunciation means not taking things up in the first place, not trying to manipulate things or force our preconceptions onto life. What we must give up is our personal will to control life. To do this we must be open, receptive and responsive to things as they are. We must be in harmony with the movement of life that clings to nothing. Renunciation is not an intended action of giving something up, but the freeing of the mind from ulterior motives. There is nothing we have to give up other than our own anxiety to control things.

—DAVID FRAWLEY

TRUE DETACHMENT

❧

Detachment is like flying high: the higher you fly, the wider a landscape you are able to view. But when you are unable to fly beyond the limited realities of your daily life, you are like a person who is confined to a narrow cell, unable to enjoy the expansion of nature. . . .

True detachment from the world becomes possible when there is increasing attachment to the Divine Self within one's heart.

—SWAMI JYOTIRMAYANANDA

CULTIVATE SIMPLICITY

❧

Sheer poverty never made anyone more peaceful; extreme but voluntary austerity is often the flip side of extravagance. The mark of successful detachment from possessions is not how few of them we have around us, but how little space they occupy in our minds.

—MAGGIE KRAMM

NONATTACHMENT IS LIBERATING

❧

Nonattachment alone leads to liberation.
All evils spring from attachment.
Therefore abandon attachment,
adhere to Reality itself, and be happy.
Even a sage can be involuntarily stirred
as a result of attachment; what then of lesser beings?

—*KULA-ARNAVA-TANTRA*

MONEY

❧

Money is the visible sign of a universal force, and this force
in its manifestation on earth works on the vital and physical
planes and is indispensable to the fullness of the outer life.
In its origin and its true action it belongs to the Divine. But
like other powers of the Divine it is delegated here and in the
ignorance of the lower Nature can be usurped for the uses of
the ego or held by Asuric [demonic] influences and per-
verted to their purpose. To reconquer it for the Divine to
whom it belongs and use it divinely for the divine life is the
supramental way for the Sadhaka [practitioner]. All wealth
belongs to the Divine and those who hold it are trustees, not
possessors.

—SRI AUROBINDO

MONEY WORSHIP

⁓

The great banks are cathedrals to money; the stock exchange is a temple. When friends once took me to a brokerage house, the lofty ceilings, the hushed tones, and air of reverence made me feel as if I were intruding on a sanctuary. Market quotations flickered across the wall like a continuous prayer, invoking bulls to protect against the bears. When the Dow went up, it lifted worshippers into an exalted state of mind; when it fell, they slipped into depression. In ancient times, devotees inhaled the smoke of burning laurel leaves or drank soma to alter states of consciousness; today we need only a digital display.

—EKNATH EASWARAN

THE SOURCE OF ALL WEALTH

∂

One day a king distributed food and other necessities to a large gathering in the courtyard of his palace. A great master joined the crowd but was turned away, because he had arrived too late that day. When the king discovered what had happened, he went to the sage and apologized profusely. He begged the master to name whatever his heart desired.

The sage responded with a question: "O king, what did you do this morning before coming to me?"

"I went to the temple."

"Why?"

"To pray to God to protect my family and the kingdom and provide ample means to distribute to the poor."

The sage smiled and said: "In that case, I don't need anything from you. I can ask God directly."

—BABA PRAKASHANANDA

9

FOOD FOR THOUGHT

‿

It has been calculated that we spend approximately seven hundred hours per year eating and drinking. Food is obviously important for sustaining the body, but it also is important to us emotionally and socially. We eat to satisfy all kinds of desires, not merely to still hunger.

For most of us, eating is associated with pleasure. If we have a problem with food, we most likely also have a problem with life as a whole, since food is symbolic of material, bodily existence.

In fact, we can regard life purely in terms of food consumption. We "eat" the world, and we are "eaten" by it. This is the essence of the ecological teaching about the "food chain"—an insight that is by no means a modern discovery, but was articulated several thousand years ago by the sages of India. Thus the *Taittiriya-Upanishad* states:

From food all creatures living on Earth are born.
On food alone they live, and into food they pass in the end.

Food should fill us with gratitude and also delight us, as the Yoga adepts are not averse to pleasure, unless they pursue a particularly rigorous ascetical path. Adherents of the more integral schools of Yoga—notably the tradition of Tantra—do not shy away from pleasure but see it as a low-level manifestation of the innate bliss (*ananda*) of our true nature, the Spirit or Self. They understand that there is nothing wrong with pleasure itself, only with our attachment to it. In fact, they endeavor to expand pleasure into bliss, and for this to be possible, you must let go of the ego, which habitually seeks to avoid pain and cling to pleasure.

Our eating habits shape us in ways few of us suspect. The food we eat is vital to both our physical and our mental health. Complementary medicine is rediscovering the close connection between body and mind, and is beginning to look at diet as a critical factor in health maintenance and restoration. Long ago, Yoga adepts provided certain rules of thumb relative to food and its consumption. In brief, we should eat wholesome food that nourishes both body and mind, and we should consume it as if we were meditating. Only then can we extract from food its most subtle essence. The material aspect of food gives nurturance on the physical level, whereas the subtle energetic aspect of food enhances our inner life by calming and elevating the mind.

THE POWER OF FOOD

❧

You are what you eat.

—POPULAR YOGA MAXIM

EAT WITH AWARENESS

❧

Remember that food is the most basic link with the source of life. Be thankful for it, pray over it, honor it. We are not just filling our belly; we are nurturing our mind and spirit as well. Eating with full awareness puts us in harmony with nature—not only with the external world, but also our own inner nature.

—CARRIE ANGUS

FOR THE YOGI COOK

All food is prepared for the Supreme, never for oneself.

Be aware of the sacred nature of all food and maintain an attitude of reverence in the same way as the gardener.

Dedicate work to the Supreme.

Make the place of work as clean and as pleasant as you can.

Keep all the utensils in good order.

Try to choose a diet that builds harmony.

Maintain a flow of loving thought during the preparation of food, in whatever way you can.

However you think during the preparation will in essence be consumed.

Realize that the food you serve, both yourself and others, will contain your love in subtle form.

—JACK SANTA MARIA

NUTRITIONAL YOGA

～

Instead of eating carelessly and hurriedly, in the midst of noise, agitation and arguments and then going off to do yoga exercises, wouldn't it be much better to understand that meals give you the perfect opportunity every day, two or three times a day, to practice relaxation, concentration and the harmonization of all the cells of your body?

—OMRAAM MIKHAËL AÏVANHOV

FOOD AND MENTAL HARMONY

～

Aside from the fact that a meal should never be eaten hurriedly, it is most important that it be taken with enjoyment, in congenial company and with pleasant surroundings. Food eaten in a state of anger, aggravation or displeasure produces a toxic condition in the body. Therefore it is better to skip a meal when in a bad state and wait until one gets back to normal.

Try to make your mealtime harmonious by avoiding upsetting discussions. A nicely set table also adds to the pleasure of eating. So does a smiling face, a cheerful word, a beautiful flower or a picture. Bless your food, and enjoy it.

—INDRA DEVI

THE DISCIPLINE OF EATING

Discipline in eating fills you with spiritual radiance. The whole purpose of this, as of all yogic disciplines, is to know God. . . .

Discipline in eating *is* a cause for celebration; therefore, accept it wholeheartedly, a little at a time. Make it yours. Let the word *discipline* become a fragrant flower for you, so that every time you hear this word you think, "Ahhh. Intoxicating! It is so wonderful!" Instead of cringing and contracting at the idea of discipline, let your being expand, let your heart run to embrace it.

—SWAMI CHIDVILASANANDA

FOOD AS MEDICINE

Food should be taken properly, as though it were
Medicine, without desire or hatred;
Not for conceit, arrogance or
Robustness, but only to maintain the body.

—NAGARJUNA

SENSUAL FASTING

A fasting of the senses is as beneficial to the mind as a light fasting of the digestive system is to the body. Meditation is a form of regular sensual fasting that can bring lasting benefits.

—JACK SANTA MARIA

DELIGHT IN THE SIMPLE THINGS

By expanding the pleasure arising from the taste of eating and drinking, one should generate a mental state filled with that delight. As a result, supreme bliss will manifest.

—*VIJNANA-BHAIRAVA*

10

MAKING PROGRESS

❧

If Yoga were designed to work on the surface only, we should expect immediate visible results. Fortunately, however, Yoga seeks to change us at all levels of existence. Its influence reaches deep into our mind. Hence we must be prepared for prolonged practice in order to allow Yoga to do its work in depth.

It is certainly possible to see positive change even after one or two sessions of yogic postures, and after six months of correct and steady postural practice, we should find ourselves calmer and more balanced. But for deep psychological and spiritual effects, we must be prepared for a lifetime of practicing Yoga in its entirety—from the moral disciplines to postures to breath control to meditation. There is no instant enlightenment. No one can enlighten or liberate us from the outside. We ourselves must do the inner work.

What is the spiritual work? It is to abandon old, fruitless patterns of behavior and thought and lay down new pathways in our brain and mind. This takes time and much effort, and we will get out of Yoga what we put into it. If all we want is a trim waistline or flexible hamstrings, we can certainly accomplish this through regular practice of the yogic postures. But if our sight is set on freeing ourselves from ignorance, unhappiness, and egotism, we must cultivate those ideals and attitudes that increase self-understanding and self-mastery, and which guide us to enlightenment, or spiritual liberation. Yoga, which is the distilled wisdom of thousands of masters, furnishes us with everything we need to succeed in such a sweeping self-transformation.

Clearly, it would be good for Yoga practitioners to learn patience and also to develop the habit of steadfast practice early on. Faith in oneself and the efficacy of Yoga are desirable as well. As the *Bhagavad-Gita* assures us: No effort on the yogic path is ever wasted. Every time we apply ourselves in the right way, we create more momentum for our spiritual journey. At a certain point, our spiritual work becomes so natural to us that everything else seems more effortful. In the long run, our entire life becomes Yoga, and we experience greater inner freedom and joy.

WE ARE OUR OWN REMEDY

Many people are unwilling to make progress on the spiritual journey because they do not want to face their desires or their fears. This is understandable. Nevertheless, if we could see how our demanding desires and blind fears, especially our fears of fear, are often the source of our sufferings, might we not take pause and reflect? This is the ironic nature of spiritual realization. As we progress spiritually, we begin to see how we, ourselves, are the primary and ultimate cause of our own sorrows. Paradoxically, this is good news! It means that we can also be the cause of our relief, our release, and our happiness.

—RON LEIFER

ON BEING SPIRITUAL

Don't be so obsessed with "being spiritual" that you cannot function effectively, nor so compulsive about satisfying desires and accomplishing personal purposes that you neglect God-remembrance.

—ROY EUGENE DAVIS

BE YOUR OWN BEST FRIEND

❧

Once we accept a bad thought it is difficult to remove it, for it enters very deeply. So be yourself, and then see yourself. This is the first step in creating amity toward yourself, and when you have amity for yourself, naturally you have amity for all. A person who does not harm himself or herself is not going to harm anybody else, for in order to harm somebody, one has to harm himself first. Think of a matchstick. When the matchstick tries to ignite something, first it must burn its own face; it is not going to burn others if it does not first burn itself.

—Munishree Chitrabhanu

GROWING MORE AND MORE AWARE

❧

In the course of spiritual growth, all of our concepts, ideas, and beliefs have to be investigated and re-evaluated over and over again. What you are thinking now may hold no value in three months or three years. You will have grown, your awareness will have increased, and your level of understanding will have risen. From being a sleepwalker, a hypnotized or conditioned person, you gradually become a person who is aware.

—Swami Sivananda Radha

KNOW YOUR TEMPERAMENT

Motivation and action vary according to temperament. Gentle people are slow to start, level-headed, and thoughtful. They are like the tortoise in the fable. Lively people are impetuous and rapid. They hurtle into action, sometimes with great vivacity, like the hare. Moderate types have an intermediate temperament, at times gentle, at times vivacious.

We can fulfill our goals by recognizing our own temperament and using it to guide our choice of profession, relationships, and leisure pursuits. The ideal is great intensity with level-headedness. We find a broad range of temperaments in the surrounding circle, in which different tendencies create richness in the group. Everybody has a chance perhaps, but it is different for each of us. That is why it is necessary to know and respect everyone's temperament and rhythm—to favor everyone's evolution and allow them to proceed at a rhythm suitable for them.

—BERNARD BOUANCHAUD

GOOD VIBRATIONS FROM
SELF-DISCIPLINE

❧

Discipline of practice is a training to gear and harmonize the external aspects of the personality, to listen to the call of something deeper within, so that the fine, subtle vibrations arising from within do not get muffled by the noises going on in our external senses and in the conscious mind.

—PANDIT USHARBUDH ARYA

REINING IN THE SENSES

❧

Just as the body is made of food, the mind is made of the sense impressions it takes in. And just as there is junk food, there are junk experiences and junk thoughts—attractively packaged, but most debilitating for the mind. Training the senses means that we need to be discriminating about what shows we watch, what music we listen to, what kinds of books and magazines we read, what kind of conversation we listen to. Every day the senses give the mind a ten-course dinner, and we can add to our *prana,* our health and vitality, by not serving it junk thoughts.

—EKNATH EASWARAN

ATTENTIVENESS

❧

A second's indiscretion or inattentiveness may bring about the ruin of treasures that have taken a lifetime to acquire. Unfailing watchfulness is the essence of Yoga life.

—SRI ANANDA ACHARYA

CENTERING

❧

It is difficult keeping the balance always. But you can't keep a balance unless you've got a center. That center is God, and if you work from that center you don't lose your way in all of the conflicting and confusing avenues which are part of life. God first.

—SRI DAYA MATA

NOBILITY

❧

Be enthusiastic about the nobleness of every man and every thing will become noble.

—SRI ANANDA ACHARYA

HOW TO BECOME TRULY BEAUTIFUL

ॐ

Learn to dress yourself with the robes of purity. Adorn yourself with the ornaments of virtues. Beautify yourself with actions that are generous and sublime. Deck your subtle body with the flowers of truthfulness, compassion, humility and cosmic love. Let your heart be a fountainsource of bliss. Thus, you will become truly beautiful.

—SWAMI JYOTIR MAYA NANDA

TIME IS PRECIOUS

ॐ

When we waste our time, it is like plucking the pearls from a dazzling necklace one by one and throwing them away. But when we use time well, each minute adds another jewel to enhance the beauty of our lives. Because time is our life, it is very precious, and we need to learn to treasure it.

—TARTHANG TULKU

CONQUERING COMPLACENCY

❧

Develop the type of personality that feels you are endlessly exploring new mystic secrets. Do not become too content with what you have accomplished in Yoga. Do not become complacent by developing the idea that you have practiced a lot of meditation and have developed wonderful qualities and have studied the scriptures. Never think that you have done all that is to be done on the spiritual path. This is a great error.

—SWAMI JYOTIRMAYANANDA

IDLENESS

❧

This is an important secret of life: if you remain idle without doing something useful your mind thinks scattered and random thoughts, and wastes its energy. Your good thoughts should definitely be brought into action. A thought is like an unripened fruit that is not yet eaten by anyone. Ripening fruit means bringing a positive thought into action. Many good thoughts die because they are not brought into action. He who is great, successful, creative, and dynamic knows how to bring all his good and creative thoughts into action, and how to give a shape and form to his creative thinking process.

—SWAMI RAMA

ENTHUSIASM

In all your actions, in all your words, in all your thoughts and feelings, be filled with enthusiasm and sing God's glory. Let your bloodstream sing the name of God, let it sing God's glory.

—SWAMI CHIDVILASANANDA

CONTROLLING NERVOUS HABITS

Look about you anywhere and you will see people tapping their feet, twiddling their fingers, twisting their mouths, chewing gum, chain-smoking, pacing restlessly, indulging helplessly in dozens of nervous habits and useless actions which merely waste the life-force so that it is not available when needed. Much of this is, of course, the expression of fear, anxiety, anger and other unhealthy mental and emotional conditions.

People who practice the self-control which Yoga teaches impart a feeling of controlled energy. They are efficient; they go about their work with a minimum of effort, with no wasted energy and few unnecessary movements. They seem to get straight to the point and are always ready to take quick, forceful action when they have to.

—RICHARD HITTLEMAN

ENERGY LEAKAGE

Energy leaks through the mouth by idle talk, gossiping, censure, scandal mongering and all sorts of useless worldly talks. . . . People do not understand the value of energy. They waste it very carelessly. They squander it like a profligate son. They repent and become weak in their old age. It is too late to gather honey in the winter.

—SWAMI SIVANANDA SARASWATI

THE TRAFFIC BODHISATTVA

When we see a red light or a stop sign, we can smile at it and thank it, because it is a bodhisattva helping us return to the present moment. The red light is a bell of mindfulness. We may have thought of it as an enemy, preventing us from achieving our goal. But now we know the red light is our friend, helping us resist rushing and calling us to return to the present moment where we can meet with life, joy, and peace. Even if you are not the driver, you can help everyone in the car if you breathe and smile.

—THICH NHAT HANH

DYNAMIC TRANQUILITY

❦

Tranquillity should not be confused with passivity or apathy. It is, rather, a dynamic quality of balance and harmony. As love is the outward flowing of energy in selflessness, and joy is the experience of accepting the natural divinity of all life, tranquillity is the experience we have when we know and accept ourselves for who and what we are.

We are the source of our own turmoil. The inner doubts, fears, impulses, the unconscious drives and motivations, all create an imbalance that leads to mental and physical suffering. We remain unaware of our spiritual identity and are caught in habits and patterns of the personality. The habits that make up this small self control us, and we bounce whenever and wherever the habits bounce, nearly always reacting to the world, with little capacity to consciously choose our actions in the world. When, through meditation, we come to experience directly our true spiritual identity, the personality with all its peaks and valleys no longer exerts a claim. We experience an inner calm and tranquillity, a center that is secure and free of conflict. From the vantage point of this calm, unattached center, we gradually resolve our inner conflicts and unfold the subtle potentials of the deeper mind.

—RUDOLPH M. BALLENTINE

HOW IMPERFECTIONS VANISH

༄

Just as the water-filled footprints
of an ox soon dry up,
so also the imperfect qualities
of a mind that is held firm
will disappear in due course.

Just as salt water turns sweet
when turned into clouds,
so also the poison of worldly objects
is turned into nectar by a firm mind
dedicated to others' welfare.

—SARAHA

SYMMETRY

༄

Your whole being should be symmetrical.
Yoga is symmetry.
That is why Yoga is a basic art.

—B.K.S. IYENGAR

II

DEALING WITH
DIFFICULTIES

ॐ

If human life were free from challenges, there could be no growth; thus we speak of "growing pains." We should not be surprised to learn that the spiritual path, which is all about growth, also presents difficulties: our resistance to change, laziness, pride, overzealousness causing bodily injury in Hatha-Yoga, mental imbalance in those branches of Yoga that work primarily through meditation, and frustration at apparently not growing fast enough.

All these hindrances are of our own making. Therefore, with the right attitude and correct practice, we also can circumvent them. Enlightenment—the goal of Yoga—happens in our own mind. That is to say, at least in part the path is as difficult as we make it for ourselves.

As we proceed in our self-transformation, we inevitably reach deeper into our own unconscious and thus have to face our shadow side. We learn to see reality as it is, without our usual projections. Then we forcefully realize that unenlightened life is indeed full of suffering. Often when this stage is reached, practitioners—out of ignorance and fear—abandon their practice. To circumnavigate these treacherous waters, we need to resort to the wise counsel of a master in the art and science of Yoga.

Every difficulty has its antidote. Therefore we should approach Yoga with great confidence. The traditional scriptures extol it as the safest ferry to liberation. But even a well-made boat needs an experienced captain to steer it clear of dangerous eddies. This is the function of mindfulness in all our activities. Whether or not we have a teacher assisting us, we always must pay attention to how we react in any given circumstance. We must be present as witness.

So long as we are on automatic, we are propelled by our own habit patterns, and this merely reproduces our state of unenlightenment. The moment we introduce mindfulness, however, we can control undesirable thoughts, motivations, emotions, and actions and activate their positive counterparts.

DIFFICULTIES ARE POTTING SOIL

Tell yourselves that disappointment and distress can serve as
a rich potting soil that will enhance the colour and scent of
your inner flowers.

—OMRAAM MIKHAËL AÏVANHOV

THE INNER OBSTACLE RACE

Remember, Yoga practice is like an obstacle race: many ob-
structions are purposely put on the way for us to pass
through. They are there to make us understand and express
our own capacities. We all have that strength, but we don't
seem to know it. We seem to need to be challenged and
tested in order to understand our own capacities. In fact,
that is the natural law. If a river just flows easily, the water in
the river does not express its power. But once you put an obstacle to the flow by constructing a dam, then you can see its
strength in the form of tremendous electrical power.

—SWAMI SATCHIDANANDA

PAIN AS TEACHER

❧

Pain is your best friend. It is infinitely more honest with you than pleasure. Despite what you might think, the painful experiences you have had benefit you far more than the pleasurable ones, even though most of us spend our lives trying to duck and hide from them. But when you can center yourself and be open to look pain dead in the eye, then you have transcended the limits of your ego and this humanity. It is then that you enter into the possibility of becoming a great being.

—SWAMI CHETANANANDA

GROWING PAINS

❧

Life is not a perpetual honeymoon. This earth is a school. Spiritual growth does not come without effort, and effort and change often means pain. I think it is meant to be that way: if there were no difficulties, we wouldn't look for anything higher. And that would be hell because it would keep us from the infinite bliss which is our birthright.

—BROTHER ANANDAMOY

LIVING IN THE WORLD

❧

If I know how to have a proper relationship with everything, everything is fine. It's my improper relationships that bring me problems, bring me enemies, likes and dislikes. But if I am neutral, no problem. And that lesson you learn only by living in the world—getting tossed, fried, roasted. You have to be fried well to become eatable. You have to be properly matured, ripened. Nobody wants to eat unripe fruit. Maturity comes only in the field. There you face challenges. Facing challenges brings you inner strength. Life is a challenge. Take a seed, put it on your altar, worship it daily, and pray, "Seed, please grow." Will it grow? No. Dig a hole, put it in there, and it gets a challenge. Then it begins to sprout.

—Swami Satchidananda

PROTECT YOURSELF WITH LIGHT

Cares and sorrows will always exist; you cannot hope to be spared, but you can deal with them if you equip yourself properly, just as we equip ourselves to deal with bad weather or mosquitoes. You protect yourself from the rain by using an umbrella, from the cold by wearing warm clothes or installing a heating system, from mosquitoes with mosquito netting or insecticide. And you can protect yourself from difficulties by looking up to a higher world and drawing down light and strength. This is the only way to overcome your difficulties.

—OMRAAM MIKHAËL AÏVANHOV

THE GRACE OF DESPAIR

꧁

If you have never reached the bottommost depths of despair, if you have not realized some point in your life at which you felt completely disintegrated, then you haven't begun your journey towards God yet. But immediately upon that disintegration, when everything you value in life is gone, there should be surrender. The cup of your personality shatters, and at that moment of shattering you surrender your will completely to the unknown, whoever the unknown is, and right there, by that very act, you have found the perfection that is God.

—PANDIT USHARBUDH ARYA

TWOFOLD GRACE

꧁

The grace of your own mind is needed to set the sail to catch the breeze of grace. God is not partial; neither is his grace conditional. He is like the magnet which draws the needle: when the needle is covered with dirt, it does not feel the attraction of the magnet. But wash away the dirt, and at once the needle feels the drawing power and becomes united with the magnet.

—SWAMI PRABHAVANANDA

THE DEEPS OF THE PATH

This path doesn't always hug the ridge tops; it often falls into deep canyons, sometimes moves along the waterways, across the valleys, deserts, and the tall peaks of your inner self. Its direction may not always seem clear as you venture into the wilderness within.

—CHARLES BREAUX

PASSING THROUGH DRY SPELLS

In gardening there are disappointments and setbacks. Sometimes the seeds fail to grow in spite of being sown in what seemed to be fertile ground. Some seeds begin to sprout almost as soon as they are put in the ground while others take their time. Yoga practice is very similar. Just when it looks as if progress is being made, something happens which points out that there is a lot more effort to be made before any result will show. There comes a feeling of dryness. Instead of a flower in the heart there is a desert of misery and frustration. This is due to the composition of the mind with its different tendencies and naturally it is impossible to live with a body and mind without having to suffer some of the problems that arise from this situation. It is no use sowing a row of lettuces and hoping that because the crop is badly needed there will be no growth of weeds when it rains and that the slugs and other creatures will go somewhere else. These things are already present in the soil and have to be dealt with as they appear. In the pattern of life they all have their function and the gardener co-operates with this pattern with understanding born of experience and without resentment. But once Yoga practice is started, the watering is taking place unseen and the seed that has been sown will surely germinate. One of the essential qualities that the gardener needs to possess is patience and another is forbearance, because he must cooperate with the vicissitudes of Nature. In the case of the Yogi gardener, he must also learn to cope with the vicissitudes of his own nature and the problems that life may bring along the way.

—JACK SANTA MARIA

REBALANCING WITH YOGA

꙳

Disease indicates that we have been making an error in terms of our lifestyle or thinking and therefore have become imbalanced. It shows us that we must make some changes if we are to live a healthy, fuller and more joyous existence. Yoga teaches us that we must learn to use and value our sufferings as springboards in our spiritual evolution. Somehow we have lost our awareness of who we are and how we should lead useful and aware lives. Loss of awareness allows disease to creep in. When we are sick, we are forced by nature to wake up to our transgressions of natural laws. Regaining our awareness through yogic practices is the key to health. The yogic process brings about rebalance, insight, understanding and appreciation of these universal, natural laws which operate in the world we live in.

—SWAMI KARMANANDA SARASWATI

DEALING WITH DIFFICULTIES
ON THE PATH

꙳

Student: Sometimes I become quite discouraged in my Sadhana [Yoga practice], and I seem to waver in my thinking and commitment. I also feel that since I have started walking the spiritual path I am facing many more trials and tribulations and even mental conflicts than ever before. Yet, I thought that Yoga was supposed to produce peacefulness and mental serenity. Can you tell me what is happening to me?

Swamiji: You are simply becoming more sensitive and paying the price for that sensitivity. Everything that is happening to you now was also happening to you before, but you were so undeveloped, so coarse in your awareness, that you were not as acutely conscious of it as you are now. Since you are becoming sensitized, you also are becoming more critical of your own life. Mistakes and failures and character flaws which you have carried all your life without caring much about them suddenly loom up clear and ugly before you, exposing themselves in the "light of your newly developed awareness." As your Sadhana develops, you will develop the quality of Sthiti Prajna, that is, the state of steady wisdom, and you will be able to see yourself and your thoughts and actions clearly without feeling either pride or disgust, pain or pleasure at the awareness. Vairagya, or detachment, rises naturally with extended Sadhana, and this detachment will allow you to view yourself without succumbing to depression and other negative emotions.

—SWAMI GITANANDA GIRI

FINDING RELIEF

෨

We often fail to get relief from disease and misery because we treat the disease and not our ignorance that has caused it.

—SHRI YOGENDRA

DON'T WORRY, BE HAPPY

෨

Discipline your personality so that you do not develop the worrying habit. You will find that when the habit infests your mind, you will worry no matter what situation you are in. You may have thought that if you were rich, you wouldn't have to worry about a thing. And then one day you become rich, and you find that your worries have multiplied along with your money.

Nothing in the world can remedy your worry except your own philosophical insight. Develop the insight that you are sustained by the Divine hand.

—SWAMI JYOTIRMAYANANDA

USING EMOTIONAL ENERGY

Confusion, tension, and depression all contain energy that can be used *for* us as well as against us. When we can calmly face our difficulties without trying to escape, without trying to manipulate or suppress our feelings, it is possible to see something that we have never seen before. We may realize very clearly that we simply do not want this pain any longer. We can then discover in ourselves the motivation to change the habits that lead us into difficulties.

We can use the energy of our emotions to skillfully cope with our problems, to rediscover the clear interplay of mind and senses that allows our energy to flow in more positive directions. Our emotions are really only energy; they become painful when we grow attached to them, and identify them as being negative. We can transform this energy into positive feelings, for ultimately, it is we ourselves who determine these reactions. The choice is up to us: we can dwell on negative emotions, or we can take their energy and use it to encourage a healthier response to our problems.

—TARTHANG TULKU

NO PROBLEM

❧

The Self has no problem. Since the Self is essentially what we are, we, too, have no real problem.

—Swami Chetanananda

12

EMBODYING
THE SPIRIT

୬

The recent wave of interest in Yoga postures appears to stem from a keen fascination with staying fit and young. We are attached to our body even when it is sick or dying. We mistakenly identify with it, whereas our true nature is the supraconscious Spirit that transcends both body and mind.

Curiously, for many—if not most—people embodiment is a real problem. I know any number of individuals who, when they first come to a session of Yoga postures and relaxation, cannot feel their feet or some other body part. Sadly, there even are a few Western Hatha-Yoga teachers who are suffering from anorexia or bulimia.

Yoga's consistent message is that we should not exclusively identify with the body, even though we ought to take proper care of it since it serves as the platform from which we can realize our true nature.

For the *yogi* and *yogini* the body is a laboratory in which pure alchemical gold (i.e., enlightenment) is produced out of base metal (i.e., the unenlightened mind). In the process, the body itself is modified. In fact, the goal of traditional Hatha-Yoga is the creation of a "diamond body" (*vajra-deha*) that is immune to aging and death. The literature of Yoga and also the oral tradition are replete with stories of masters who have succeeded in "cheating death."

In his groundbreaking book *The Future of the Body,* Michael Murphy has collected a massive amount of data about the body's astounding potential that removes at least some of the claims made by Yoga from the realm of fantasy. Modern gene research, too, is holding out the possibility of extraordinary health and longevity. Perhaps sometime in the future, genetic engineering and Yoga will meet on common ground. Certainly the wisdom of Yoga will be necessary to prevent the specter of an out-of-control biotechnology.

However much we may be able to increase our physical strength and flexibility, augment our body's health and beauty, or extend our lifespan, we still have to face the fact that the wellspring of happiness lies not in the material realm but in the spiritual dimension of our being. It is the realization of who we truly are that infuses everything else with meaning. So long as we are obsessed with our body (or our mind), the ego is intact, which means that we are estranged from our true Self, and thus genuine happiness and freedom elude us.

When we have realized our ultimate nature, the omnipresent Spirit, we discover that we are the eternal background of all bodies—past, present, and future. We tend to be so anxious about losing our present body, whereas the truth of the matter is that all bodies—including the present one—are continually arising in the Spirit.

BE FRIENDLY TOWARD YOUR BODY

Do not fight your body. Do not carry the world on your shoulders like Atlas. Drop that heavy load of unnecessary baggage and you will feel better.

Do not kill the instinct of the body for the glory of the pose. Do not look at your body like a stranger, but adopt a friendly approach toward it. Watch it, listen to it, observe its needs, its requests, and even have fun. Play with it as children do, sometimes it becomes very alert and swift.

To be sensitive is to be alive.

—Swami Karmananda Saraswati

IN YOUR OWN IMAGE

In a very literal sense, the body is a living sculpture of yourself. Aside from genetic inheritance and the body images received in childhood, the body is molded by changes in the psychological state. Thoughts and feelings as psychic energy in the aura affect the physical body via nerve centers and endocrine glands, altering its apparent structure and function. Some examples of this are: the drastic physical changes in appearance which are clearly seen in people subject to multiple personalities, and the superhuman strength experienced in emergencies or under hypnosis.

—Charles Breaux

YOU ARE NOT THE BODY

୬

We look at our bodies and, since we see something contained by unbroken skin that looks like one thing, we say, "Well, this is what I am." Much of our attention is then taken up by our experiences of the body and its processes. It gets born, it grows up, it ages. It engages in activity and it rests. It gets sick and it feels healthy. It generates children and feels the pain of loss. It is always with us. We get up, we look at it every morning in the mirror, we hit it, we feel it, it complains to us if we don't treat it right. Consequently, we think we have something that we can call "my body"—"me." In fact, however, it is not. This is not *you* that you are sitting in, but just a group of cells.

—SWAMI CHETANANANDA

THE BODY IS AN AIRPLANE

The body is like an airplane, inside which is seated the pilot and Self, captain and master. Mindstuff is like the engine of the airplane, and senses are like wings. By means of this airplane of body and mind, Self flies peacefully and carefully over mountains, rivers, and valleys of problems. As radar and searchlights and constant communication are supplied to guide the pilot, so in meditation constant information, suggestion, and guiding hints are manifested by Nature. These are light, sound current, and other things. If constant attention is given, this airplane will reach its destination successfully. As a pilot opposes gravity, a small mistake may give gravitational forces a chance to create an accident. Likewise a small mistake in vigilance may offer a chance to gravitational forces of drives and desires to cause an accident of mental forces by throwing them into the ocean and mountains of sensual delights.

—RAMMURTI S. MISHRA

YOUR BODY IS YOUR CHILD

❧

Your body must be disciplined like a child, calmly but forcefully. You are, in fact, reeducating your body and as the various areas are convinced that you are serious (just like the
child), they will begin to obey.

—RICHARD HITTLEMAN

MY BODY, MY TEACHER

❧

The body is a teacher of mine,
being the cause of dispassion and discernment and
being subject to birth and death,
which always are attendant with pain.
Even though it has a different destiny from my own,
with its help I ponder the principles of existence
and move about free from attachment.

—*UDDHAVA-GITA*

FEELING THE WHOLE BODY

A powerful but simple practice is to try to maintain presence in the body continuously throughout the day. Feel the body as a whole. The mind is worse than a crazed monkey, jumping from one thing to the next; it has a hard time focusing on one thing. But the body is a source of experience more stable and constant, and using it as an anchor for awareness will help the mind to grow calmer and more focused. Just as the participation of the mind is essential in organizing and nourishing the physical aspects of life, the mind needs the body in order to stabilize in calm presence, which is fundamentally important to all practices.

—TENZIN WANGYAL RINPOCHE

THE BODY'S TRUTH

※

In the final analysis, we can control only ourselves. But we are often dismayed at our inability to master even this. What prevents us? When we feel out of control, it is usually because there is a conflict between what we think and what we feel. Our feelings may scream one thing while our minds demand something else. But our bodies, which are the storage units for our feelings, simply cannot lie. Whatever we feel in our bodies is our truth.

—JUDITH LASATER

GOOD HEALTH

※

Good health is more than feeling physically and mentally well. It means that one is whole spiritually, that one feels good, sometimes in spite of what's going on in the body.

—BROTHER ACHALANANDA

DISHARMONY AND ILL HEALTH

❧

Every jerk of disharmony, every little sign of ill health, every trifle deviation from the normal rhythm of healthful living on the various planes of consciousness, even though it may not show any immediate evil effect, does not fail to leave a permanent mark upon one's health on the debit side. Such little acts and feelings of disharmony, besides producing ill health, deduct more from the years of life and complete living than anything else and, to a great extent, make life a failure and a burden instead of a benefaction and pleasure.

—SHRI YOGENDRA

BODILY SURRENDER

❧

Shake the container and the contents spill. Move the body and the mind loses concentration. Force the body to stay still and it rebels. Teach the body to surrender; relax your muscles and nerves; let go of them from your mind; the mind becomes free of the bondage of the flesh. This is the surrender of the body to the mind, and the mind will continue to take care of the body without catering to its every whim.

—PANDIT USHARBUDH ARYA

SITTING STILL

People began doing postures so they could sit for a long time. And what will happen if you sit longer? Conflicts will disappear. You will feel calm. So learn to sit first before you talk about meditation.

—VIJAYENDRA PRATAP

UNDER YOUR OWN STEAM

The purpose of deliberate restraint and controlled relaxation is to confine tensions to their places where they can work constructively and not allow the energy of the body to dribble wastefully away in unnecessary motion. You should keep your steam in to run your own engine and not permit it to escape and befog your mind or cloud the lives of others.

—MARCIA MOORE AND MARK DOUGLAS

THE BENEFITS OF RELAXATION

When we are relaxed, calm and open like a pool in a glade, the quality of our inner nature stands out clearly. We have a keen and direct perception of ourselves and our interaction with everything that is going on around us. Our energy is well-focused; we can think clearly, and we are able to plan and organize our thoughts effectively. We are self-assured: we know what we want to accomplish, what our obstacles are, and how to dissolve them. We work with ease, moving fluidly, in tune with our work rather than resisting its requirements, simply doing what needs to be done. Our work takes on a vital texture, alive with challenge and fulfillment, and the results of our actions reflect the relaxed quality we bring to them.

—TARTHANG TULKU

BE LIKE A TREE

You must be firmly rooted. Such is the first law. Then grow and assert yourself. At this moment open yourself, stretch out your arms to feel your radiation around you, and then bring the universe back to you with your head held high, for it touches the sun. Be deep, wide, tall, truly a Tree of Life.

—LIZELLE REYMOND

ANTIGRAVITY YOGA

❧

When the abandonment to gravity comes into action, resistance ceases, fear vanishes, order is regained, nature starts again to function in its natural rhythm and the body is able to blossom fully, allowing the river of life to flow freely through all its parts.

—Vanda Scaravelli

ASANA

❧

The body is my temple
and asanas are my prayers.

While practicing asanas,
learn the art of adjustment.

When your posture is imbalanced,
the practice is physical;
balanced asanas lead to spiritual practice.

As a goldsmith weighs gold,
you have to adjust your body so that it is
perfectly balanced in the median plane.

As pearls are held on a thread,
all the limbs should be held
on the thread of intelligence.

If your body *can* do more and you do not do it,
that is unethical practice.

Ethical discipline of the asana is
when you extend correctly, evenly
and to the maximum.

The brain is the hardest part of the body
to adjust in asanas.

If the brain is silent but attentive
while performing asanas,
your practice is nonviolent.

—B.K.S. IYENGAR

13

THE BREATH OF LIFE

Thousands of years ago, the masters of Yoga realized that the breath is the "missing link" between the body and mind. This simple insight is the key to transforming both the body and the mind, for by regulating the breath we can influence the nervous system and the brain.

Yogis have shown amazing control even over autonomic nervous system functions such as heartbeat, pulse, digestion, metabolism, and skin temperature. For example, Swami Rama, founder of the Himalayan International Institute in Pennsylvania, demonstrated control over his brain's electrical output. He was able to induce delta waves characteristic of sleep while remaining fully conscious.

The Sanskrit word for "breath" is *prana,* which also means "life." Thus *prana* could be translated as "the breath of life." This corresponds to the Chinese *chi* (or Japanese *ki*), which is widely known in the West through the martial arts of the Far East. Martial arts practitioners know how to pack the body with life force in order to deliver lethal blows or prevent injury in a fight, or even to heal themselves and others when injury has occurred.

Breath is the outer aspect of *prana,* which, according to

Yoga, is a subtle kind of energy sustaining the body. Yoga has developed many techniques for controlling breath known as *pranayama*. This Sanskrit word is composed of two terms, namely *prana* and *ayama*, the latter meaning "lengthening." Thus *pranayama* is the expansion of the life force in the body through regulation of the breath. As we deepen and harmonize our breathing, we also slow it down. This, in turn, slows down, or calms, our nervous system (through activation of the parasympathetic nervous system), which directly impacts on the brain and obliges our mind to slow down as well.

As we become calmer, our mind also becomes more lucid and the flow of our awareness is less and less interrupted by intruding thoughts and emotions. Here we enter the territory of meditation and higher states of consciousness.

It is no accident that the Latin words *spiritus* and *anima* signify both "breath" and "spirit." The same is true of the Greek term *pneuma* and the Sanskrit word *atman*. For the breath is the royal road to the Spirit. Breath control is the fourth limb of Patanjali's eightfold path and is followed by sensory inhibition, concentration, meditation, and ecstasy. From the state of ecstatic unification it is but a small leap into freedom.

BREATH IS FOREMOST

The best and the greatest is breath.

—*Brihad-Aranyaka-Upanishad*

THE BREATH OF LIFE

Breath is life. And life is breath. So long as the breath remains in the body, so long there is life. Hence by means of the breath one attains immortality in this world.

—*Kaushitaki-Upanishad*

THE BREATH IS THE WATER OF LIFE

Our breath is constantly rising and falling, ebbing and flowing, entering and leaving our bodies. Full body breathing is an extraordinary symphony of both powerful and subtle movements that massage our internal organs, oscillate our joints, and alternately tone and release all the muscles in the body. It is a full participation with life.

—*Donna Farhi*

BECOME A VESSEL FOR LIFE

Breathing is one of the simplest things in the world. We breathe in, we breathe out. When we breathe with real freedom, we neither grasp for nor hold on to the breath. No effort is required to pull the breath in or to push the breath out. Given the simplicity of breathing one would think it was the easiest thing to do in the world. However, if it were truly so easy there would be few unhappy or unhealthy people in the world. To become a welcome vessel for the breath is to live life without trying to control, grasp, or push away. And how easy is this? The process of breathing is the most accurate metaphor we have for the way that we personally approach life, how we live our lives, and how we react to the inevitable changes that life brings us.

—DONNA FARHI

INHALING ENERGY

✧

There are those who inhale and exhale the breath but do not take in energy and there are those who take in a lot of energy in just a few breaths. You must have training in the practice of unifying yourself with the energy when you breathe in the air. This is the secret of Yoga, the very essence. Inhalation and exhalation are only the mechanical parts of the practice, the outer form.

—Vimala Thakar

BREATHING AS CONSCIOUS PRACTICE

✧

Every breath can be a practice. With the inhalation, imagine drawing in pure, cleansing, relaxing energies. And with each exhalation, imagine expelling all obstacles, stress, and negative emotions. This is not something that requires a particular place in which to sit. It can be done when in the car on the way to work, waiting for a stop light, sitting in front of the computer, preparing a meal, cleaning the house, or walking.

—Tenzin Wangyal Rinpoche

TRUE BREATH CONTROL

༄

Breath control is the conviction that this entire universe is false.

—*Laghu-Avadhuta-Upanishad*

THE WAVE OF THE BREATH

༄

So when the breath is observed, it is not an act induced in the mind by something other than the mind, but rather it is the very wave of the mind, like a tide flowing and ebbing into a bay, into a channel going out from the sea. Imagine a lake under the dome of your skull from which these waves are going out, but at the moment this lake is not a lake, it's a witch's cauldron bubbling all over the place. Bubble here, bubble, bubble, bubble there. But when the meditational process begins, you take the lake and you let the tide flow into a channel. So you observe the breath as a wave of the mind flowing, a wave of the mind ebbing and a wave of the mind flowing, a wave of the mind ebbing and flowing. You are not watching this from outside but from the very center of the composition of the mind from where you are sending the waves and bringing the waves back and sending the waves and bringing the waves back.

—Swami Veda Bharati

MINDFUL BREATHING

We spend most of our time caught up in memories of the past or looking ahead to the future, full of worries and plans. The breath has none of that "other-timeness." When we truly observe the breath, we are automatically placed in the present. We are pulled out of the morass of mental images and into a bare experience of the here-and-now. In this sense, breath is a living slice of reality. A mindful observation of such a miniature model of life itself leads to insights that are broadly applicable to the rest of our experience.

—Henepola Gunaratana

FLOW

When the practice of postures is combined with conscious breathing and deep states of concentration and absorption, *prana* will sometimes spontaneously "take over" the practice. Suddenly, energy itself will begin to direct the flow of postures. In these moments we may have a sense of effortlessness, of complete surrender to a force greater than ourselves. This experience can be surprising, compelling, and blissful. And, it appears to be completely out of our control. We cannot make it happen. We can only let it happen.

—Stephen Cope

RELAXING WITH THE BREATH

The image of relaxing in a boat tethered in restless waters is an interesting metaphor for the process of breath awareness, which is a kind of mental mooring. When you rest your attention on the breath, your awareness is anchored. Currents and crosscurrents of thinking continue to create sensations of movement in the mind, but a steady focus on breathing prevents these mental provocations from disturbing your equilibrium. . . .

When the Greek hero Odysseus sailed past the island of the Sirens—the voices of sensual desires that called out to passing ships—he lashed himself to the mast of his vessel before he came within earshot. Like Odysseus, you must lash yourself to the mast of your breath.

—ROLK SOVIK

BREATHING AWAY FEAR

Let us observe ... the way a nervous or anxious man breathes. Such a man does not venture to breathe out fully, he does not dare to empty his lungs and remain at peace until the moment when the in-breathing phase comes of itself. This is a symptom of deep fear and anxiety. When the lungs are empty an anxious man is in dread of the void, and he gives himself over to the movement of breathing in so as to recover his habitual feeling of life and a state of passing relief.

But in the case of a healthy man, that is, a man who is perfectly harmonized, in agreement with himself and the cosmos, breathing has a metaphysical significance, it is the symbol of the rhythm of exchange between the individual and his principle. Each breathing out expresses an entire surrendering of the creature to God and each inspiration signifies the return of the divine influx.

Between the two moments, at the moment when the lungs are empty, the unmanifested divine is approached. Thus we can see how fear hinders us from being and experiencing the formless.

—JEAN KLEIN

14

LOVE, SEX,
AND BEYOND

Ultimately, everything boils down to whether or not we can love unconditionally. At least this is one way of describing the spiritual path.

What we commonly call love is often little more than a sentimental emotion peppered with a good dose of self-interest. The situation is still less appealing when we consider sexual love. In practice, sex and love can be almost mutually exclusive, though they need not be. Love is a matter of the heart, which in yogic terms is the fourth of seven major psychospiritual centers (*cakras*) of the body.

By contrast, the sexual impulse is anchored in the second center, which is located at the genitals. If we can engage in sex with an awakened heart, sexual *love* is indeed a possibility, but our culture deemphasizes the heart and overemphasizes sex. Surveys have shown that adult men and women are preoccupied with sex and sexual fantasies throughout the day. Today American children start having intercourse at the age of fourteen and younger, when they still lack emotional maturity. By the time they reach adulthood, they feel jaded and their lives are devoid of meaning.

Since ancient times, Yoga masters have recommended

sexual abstinence (called *brahmacarya*) during the first twenty-one years of one's life. During this time, children and adolescents learn to properly harness the awesome power of libido. Then, as adults, they are not ruled by the second *cakra* but engage in intercourse in a wholesome, balanced fashion as an expression of mutural respect and love.

For many people, sex is mere entertainment—a diversion from boredom and everyday anxiety and frustration. The problem is that it proffers only a trickle of pleasure, which cannot satisfy us deeply, whereas our potential is for unimaginable bliss (*ananda*). We use sexual gratification as a substitute for real happiness, and because it is neither profound nor lasting, we return to sexual stimulation over and over again like addicts. At least this is the perspective of Yoga.

Yoga is not opposed to pleasure, only to our enslavement to it. It also recognizes that the enjoyment we derive from our senses or the mind is nothing by comparison with our innate bliss. When we are in touch with our true nature, everything we experience is filled with delight, as bliss eclipses both pleasure and pain.

In Tantra-Yoga, India's great spiritual masters have developed an approach that values embodiment and therefore also assigns an appropriate place to pleasure, including sexual pleasure. Tantra-Yoga is, however, sadly misunderstood and misrepresented in the West. Contrary to the pop versions of this 1,500-year-old tradition, the adepts of traditional Tantra-Yoga seek bliss, not orgasm; liberation, not an improved sex life. Tantra-Yoga endeavors to strike a balance between self-discipline and spontaneity, and between Self-realization and living an active life in the world.

The yogic path demands of us that we transmute ourselves at all levels. It is not enough to restrain our thoughts; we must also rid ourselves of negative emotions and cultivate positive emotions like love, compassion, and kindness toward all beings. This involves regulating our sexual impulse and using that energy to fulfill our spiritual destiny.

LOVE IS RADIANCE

❧

Love is the Sacrifice. Love is the Law. Love is Radiance, not Contraction. Love is the action in which ego and all reactions are dissolved, since all such things are only contraction. Fear is only contraction. Sorrow is only contraction. Anger is only contraction. Mind in all of its realms, high or low, is only contraction. Where contraction ceases, there is no ego to survive, no reactions to dramatize into separation, no fear, no sorrow, no anger, no thought, no other.

—BUBBA FREE JOHN (ADI DA)

LOVE AND HAPPINESS

❧

In Love, God is found in the world, and the world is found in God. And for the glory of God to be experienced, happiness has to increase.

—MAHARISHI MAHESH YOGI

LOVE IS BLIND

Negative intentions evaporate
beneath the rising sun of Love.
All sense of animosity disappears.
Who is enemy and who is friend
when only Love shines?

—SRI RAMAKRISHNA

LOVE IS ALL THERE IS

When there is neither desire nor fear, there is but love.

—JEAN KLEIN

THE CRADLE OF LOVE

When emotions are purified they develop into love, which is an
important step in the awakening of further levels of consciousness. Feelings which have been purified bring us into the presence
of the Divine and from the Divine we feel a sense of protection.

—SWAMI SIVANANDA RADHA

THE RECIPROCITY OF LOVE

For creatures who want to be loved, appreciated, even adored, we certainly go about fulfilling our desire in a curiously unfulfilling way. Instead of manufacturing it ourselves in the little love machine inside our chests, we complain about not getting enough of it, search frantically for someone else to give it to us, and try to make ourselves more lovable by improving our looks or earning more money. But the truth is, the Beatles song has it right. The love you take is equal to the love you make. In other words, the most effective way to get love is to generate it yourself.

By cultivating caring, loving feelings you can actually provide yourself with the nourishment you seek. At the same time, by radiating those feelings outward to others, you can touch their tender hearts and naturally elicit the same feelings in them, creating a flow of love that keeps circulating between you and building on itself.

—STEPHAN BODIAN

BOUNDLESS LOVE

True love is boundless like the ocean and, rising and swelling within one, spreads itself out and, crossing all boundaries and frontiers, envelops the whole world.

—"MAHATMA" M. K. GANDHI

THE LAW OF LOVE

The most ancient traveler in the world is called love. Even before this earth came into existence, that omnipotent and omniscient power called truth expanded to create the universe because of love. Love means expansion. And then there is its opposite, called hatred or contraction. Watch what happens some day when you start hating somebody—when someone is not doing what you want, is not fulfilling your expectations. You contract your personality, you isolate yourself. So there are two laws of life: the law of expansion, and the law of contraction.

—Swami Rama

LOVE AND SEX

Sex is a sensation. Love is a state of being, a lasting relationship which we can slowly make permanent. That is the deepest desire in all of us, to make this state of union permanent.

—Eknath Easwaran

TRUE LOVE

❧

We expect our wives or husbands or children to make us happy by behaving the way our ego desires. We all want others to make us feel important, wise, and attractive. So we spend twenty to fifty years living together—expecting and demanding many things from each other—but this has nothing to do with experiencing our love and walking on the real spiritual path.

When we truly love someone, we love the Light within that person. The process of enlightenment is the path of learning to appreciate the Light within both ourselves and those we love, and seeking to allow the full expression of our Self as well as the Self of others.

—SWAMI RAMA

IGNITING LOVE

When the force and power of all our desires can be channeled toward the Divine, rather than toward attaining the charms of the external world, then love, the strongest force in the universe, leads its energy to the path. That loves exists within all, and can be experienced when the mind is no longer dissipated by the ego and the objects of the senses. When the spark of that love is ignited, it can create a burning desire to experience union with the Absolute. That flame is capable of burning away all the little desires of life, until only one flame exists—the flame of devotion that burns eternally in the chamber of the heart.

—BHOLE PRABHU

DEVOTION

Like a cloud drifting in the sky,
Devotion pours down showers of bliss.
He whose mind gets filled like a reservoir
reaps the entire fruit of his birth, none other.

—SHANKARA

WHO LOVES THE LORD?

❧

Even if one lives in the world, one must go into solitude now and then. It will be of great help to a man if he goes away from his family, lives alone, and weeps for God even for three days. Even if he thinks of God for one day in solitude, when he has the leisure, that too will do him good. People shed a whole jug of tears for wife and children. But who cries for the Lord?

—SRI RAMAKRISHNA

TRUE LOVE TRANSFORMS

❧

The highest understanding of love lies in its power to transform lives, restore health, and bring about a sense of total well-being. It is the other end of the spectrum which is directed by desire—the limited, contracted form of love—that has a tremendously destructive potential.

—SWAMI CHETANANDA

RISING ABOVE SEX

You have to rise above sex—not wrestle with it, but rise above it. Because, if you do not have an overall concentrated urge or ambition in life, then the clamour of these little senses becomes a great din in your life. Your life will always be under that clamour. But, if you have got an overwhelming urge for something else, then this clamour does not reach you at all, because you are too busy engaging your entire attention in some other direction.

—SWAMI CHIDANANDA

THE LANGUAGE OF LOVE

The most ancient language in the world is the language of love. This language doesn't lie or misinform or distort the world, unlike the other languages we use for manners or politeness. The words of other languages become empty; those empty words have nor heart or love.

—SWAMI RAMA

LOVE AND NONATTACHMENT

With love there is no painful reaction; love brings only a reaction of bliss. If it does not, it is not love; it is a mistaking of
something else for love. When you have succeeded in loving
your husband, your wife, your children, the world, the whole
universe, in such a manner that there is no reaction of pain
or jealousy, no selfish feeling, then you are in a fit state to be
unattached. . . .

To attain this nonattachment is almost a life-work; but as
soon as we have reached this point we have attained the goal
of love and become free.

—SWAMI VIVEKANANDA

CHASTE LOVE

There is only one way to be chaste if chastity is not to be negative, and that is, to love deeply.

—LEWIS THOMPSON

15

GREAT REALIZATIONS
IN SMALL THINGS

Yogis and *yoginis* regard life as a school. The principal lesson that we are expected to learn is that we are the same One, the singular Being-Consciousness-Bliss, which is known as *atman* or *brahman* in the Sanskrit language. When we fail to learn this truth, we must repeat the class. Yoga calls this reincarnation—a teaching found in many other traditions as well, including early Christianity and Judaism.

We do not need to believe in reincarnation (the repeated assumption of a new body) to practice Yoga, but many great minds have found this teaching eminently plausible. Among their ranks we find people like Pythagoras, Socrates, Schopenhauer, Goethe, William Blake, Ralph Waldo Emerson, Wordsworth, Tennyson, and Whitman. Whatever our own view on this may be, to succeed on the yogic path we must see ourselves in the larger context of life. Then we realize that life gives us countless opportunities for self-inspection and self-understanding, which are essential preliminaries to self-transcendence and self-transformation. Without these four, ultimate Self-realization is impossible.

We are able to look at ourselves critically because of our innate witnessing capacity, which is a fundamental characteristic of the Spirit, of Self. As Yoga affirms, we are free even now, but our own mind obscures this great truth from us. Hence we must polish the mirror of the mind to see clearly. The more we behold the One in everything, the greater are our freedom and happiness.

We do not have to shun the world, as has been the custom of ascetics, but we must allow the light of the spirit to transmute it. We can do this by lifting ourselves by the means of Yoga and inviting the Spirit to illumine our mind. Then our thoughts, emotions, and actions will conform to our higher nature, enabling us to radically transfigure our body and the world around us.

Long before we are finally liberated or enlightened, however—and we must be prepared for the long haul—we contribute to the transformation of the world. As Sage Patanjali makes clear in his *Yoga-Sutra*, compiled roughly two millennia ago, the adept who has gained self-mastery activates all kinds of extraordinary abilities. For instance, in the presence of a *yogi* or *yogini* who has mastered the virtue of nonharming, even the most ferocious wild animals may become peaceful. Or, to give another example, when an adept is firmly grounded in the virtue of truthfulness, his or her word will always come true.

With the exception of adepts who have chosen to live in total solitude in a remote forest or mountain cave, Yoga masters have always been a support and beacon of light and hope for people. They have acted as counselors and healers, and their company is typically sought by hundreds and sometimes hundreds of thousands.

Self-realization is preceded by many smaller realizations, or insights, all of which are important on the yogic path. We ought to stay open to them and receive them gratefully. In this way, we can gradually make ourselves transparent to the Light and then spread it to everyone else.

LIVING YOGA

In the right view both of life and of Yoga, all life is either
consciously or subconsciously a Yoga.

—Sri Aurobindo

LIBERATION NOW

Why think of liberation at some future time?
Liberation is in the little things, here and now.

—B.K.S. Iyengar

TRUTH IS HERE

Truth is not far away; it is ever present. It is not something to
be attained since not one of your steps leads away from it.

—Dogen

CONTENTMENT

We must live in the now to follow the path to enlightenment. In the lower realms of the mind, where time and space
seem very real, we are worried about the past or concerned
about the future. These two intermingle and limit conscious
awareness. A person functioning in the now is in control of
his own mind. He is naturally happier, more successful. He is
performing every task with his fullest attention, and the re-
wards are to be seen equally in the quality of his work and
the radiance of his face. He cannot be bored with anything
he does, however simple or mundane. Everything is interesting, challenging, fulfilling. A person living fully in the now is
a content person.

—SATGURU SIVAYA SUBRAMANIYASWAMI

OPENNESS

The openness to Life Itself that we cultivate frees us from a
great deal of conditioning and many inherent, and inherited,
assumptions. . . . Life is not about answers. It *is* about learning to live in the middle of complete uncertainty, and doing
so gracefully.

—SWAMI CHETANANANDA

EMBRACING LIFE

You must learn to welcome consciously the most unexpected events of life, to be entirely transparent in front of them, without any motive, either right or wrong. At that moment avoid all judgment, for you do not know what law is in operation.

—LIZELLE REYMOND

SEEING BEAUTY EVERYWHERE

Yoga teaches that beauty is everywhere if one can learn to see it, and that complete concentration upon a beautiful thought, scene or object will result in relaxation of the mind and achievement of tranquillity.

—NANCY PHELAN AND MICHAEL VOLIN

BATHING IN BEAUTY

Every day you should dip your soul into beauty. Meditation is the means to see beauty in the soul, which is the source of all beauty.

—HARI PRASAD SHASTRI

TASTING THE SWEETNESS
IN EVERYONE

❧

Sweetness. This entire universe is filled with sweetness. God wants us to experience this sweetness, to melt in this honey-like sweetness by having sweet thoughts, by speaking sweet words, by performing sweet actions, by letting the sweetness from our soul flow into other hearts. Every heart is made of sweetness. Sweetness is another name for the heart.

—SWAMI CHIDVILASANANDA

CONVERSING WITH NATURE

❧

Smile with the flowers and green grass.
Play with the birds and the deer.
Shake hands with the ferns and twigs.
Talk to the rainbow, wind, stars and the sun.
Converse with the running brook
And the waves of the sea.
Develop friendship with all your neighbours,
Dogs, cats, trees and flowers.
Then you will have a wide, perfect and full life.

—SWAMI SIVANANDA SARASWATI

THE EYES OF THE SOUL

꙳

It does not require a large eye to see a large mountain. The reason is that, though the eye is small, the soul which sees through it is greater and vaster than all the things which it perceives. In fact, it is so great that it includes all objects, however large or numerous, within itself. For it is not so much that you are within the cosmos as that the cosmos is within you.

—MEHER BABA

INSPIRATION

꙳

The mind requires daily inspiration. The conception behind the word "inspiration" is "something breathed in from above," not from the physical sky but infused transcendentally into a man's mind: something good, beautiful and true, giving guidance to each individual in his walk of life.

—HARI PRASAD SHASTRI

ENTHUSIASM, THE SECRET
OF ETERNAL YOUTH

Youth is not a time of life—it is a state of mind. It is not a matter of ripe cheeks, red lips and supple knees. It is a temper of the will, a quality of the imagination, a vigor of the emotions. It is freshness of the deep springs of life. Nobody grows old by merely living a number of years. People grow old only by deserting their ideals. Years wrinkle the skin, but to give up enthusiasm wrinkles the soul.

—SWAMI BUA, AGE 110

PEACE IS OUR GREATEST GIFT

Peace is a natural mind-state in every one of us. Peace has been there since the day we were born and it is going to be there till the day we die. It is our greatest gift; so why do we think we have no peace of mind?

Experiencing peace is like looking at our hands. Usually, we see only the fingers—not the spaces in between. In a similar manner, when we look at the mind, we are aware of the active states, such as our running thoughts and the one-thousand-and-one feelings that are associated with them, but we tend to overlook the intervals of peace between them.

—THYNN THYNN

SEEING REALITY WITH A CALM MIND

༄

When the mind is calm, it does not create a wall between you and the Reality, and you can then see the Reality face to face. That is called God. God is the center of power, life, light, and love.

—SWAMI RAMA

SPIRITUAL BLINDNESS

༄

The saints say that the world is blind. A blind man may be defined as a person who cannot see what is present before him. God is omnipresent, and yet we are not aware of His august presence. The saints are aware that He is present in every particle of this universe. Their eyes are open. But we do not perceive Him and therefore we are accounted blind. The human body is the temple of the living God. He resides within this house of clay. But when we close our eyes, we are conscious of nothing but darkness within. Saints explain that this darkness is that of ignorance. We lack real wisdom. The true Light does not shine within us. Hence the darkness in which our mind is enshrouded.

—MAHARAJ CHARAN SINGH

BEYOND STRUGGLE

❧

Your work really begins when you release struggle. To let go of struggle initiates a change of vibration within you. This change puts you in touch with the flow of Life Itself, which is essentially what you are. To cultivate your awareness of this flow is your real work.

When you're in touch with the flow of Life and feel your heart and mind open, you'll note that a certain presence starts to assert itself. This presence changes your physical chemistry, your feelings, and your mind. It is the spirit itself, starting to inform you about yourself, about it, about Life, and about God. It's a simple work.

—SWAMI CHETANANANDA

PERFECT SILENCE

❧

Thus, only true Silence is eternal speech, the one word *om* (inner sound), the Heart-to-Heart talk. Silence is the true advice. It is the perfect advice. It is suited only for the most advanced seeker. Others are unable to draw full inspiration from it. Therefore, they require words to explain Truth.

—SWAMI SATYESWARANANDA GIRI

BEING PRESENT

၃

I am therefore
you are
In the present
Of the present
we are.

—GURANI ANJALI

DEATH IS A BEGINNING

၃

Death is not an end, but a new beginning. Under the stress of conflicting passions and earthly desires, biological cravings and love of pleasure and power, is hidden an eternal stream of pure consciousness which is not affected by the law of cause and effect and which is ever tranquil bliss and freedom, real love and truth. This is the real Self of man.

—HARI PRASAD SHASTRI

THE UNIMPORTANCE OF DEATH

୬

Death is unimportant to a yogi; he does not mind when he is going to die. What happens after death is immaterial to him. He is only concerned with life—with how he can use his life for the betterment of humanity.

—B.K.S. IYENGAR

ALL IS BRAHMAN

୬

The world is a picture gallery. The Lord has painted the spring and the autumn, joys and disappointments, sufferings and exaltations, on the canvas of time-space. Let us be witnesses and let us enjoy the creation of the ever-blissful Lord.

We will not possess or appropriate any of the pictures, nor apply personal feelings to them. Each must remind us of the master hand of the Divine Painter. We enjoy the world as the divine sport. Our minds and egos are also pictures.

There is no room for selection, acceptance or rejection. All is Brahman.

—HARI PRASAD SHASTRI

DISCOVERING THE SUBTLEST
OF THE SUBTLEST

৩০

Long ago, Sage Uddalaka Aruni sought to instruct his beloved son Shvetaketu in the wisdom about the ultimate Self.

Sage Uddalaka said: "Bring me the fruit of that fig tree."

Shvetaketu said: "Here it is, Sire."

Sage Uddalaka: "Break it open."

Shvetaketu: "It is broken, Sire."

Sage Uddalaka: "What do you see?"

Shvetaketu: "There are very small seeds, Sire."

Sage Uddalaka: "Break one of them open."

Shvetaketu: "It is broken, Sire."

Sage Uddalaka: "What do you see?"

Shvetaketu: "Nothing much, Sire."

Sage Uddalaka: "Beloved son, the subtle essence that you can no longer discern is the source of that fig tree. Believe me. Likewise, the subtle essence behind this universe is Truth. That is the Self. And that are you!"

—*CHANDOGYA-UPANISHAD*

16

MEDITATION
AND PRAYER

❧

Meditation is the principal means by which most branches of Yoga lead us to liberation. Even Karma-Yoga, the Yoga of self-transcending action, calls for mindfulness during all one's daily activities. Meditation, as commonly understood, is simply mindfulness while being seated in a stable and tension-free posture.

In Patanjali's eightfold path (see page 44), meditation is the sixth limb. It follows upon concentration (*dharana*) and leads to ecstasy (*samadhi*), which, in turn, is the portal to liberation. While concentration trains the quicksilver mind to abide in one place, meditation builds on that facility to connect with the deepest or highest part of our being.

Prayer, like meditation, has traditionally been used for the same purpose. It extends from verbal prayer, in which we speak to the Divine as if it were apart from us, to silent prayer, which is peaceful waiting or abiding. Many Western Yoga practitioners do not know that *yogis* and *yoginis* have traditionally availed themselves of prayer to deepen their meditation and spiritual life. Especially in Bhakti-Yoga, the path of devotional self-surrender to a higher principle, prayer is widely employed as a conduit for divine grace.

Admittedly, most forms of Yoga subscribe to a nondualist metaphysics ("There is only the One, which manifests in countless ways"). But so long as we have not actually realized this ultimate singular Reality, we continue to move in the realm of apparent multiplicity: We experience ourselves as separate from everything else, and this sense of separation makes us insecure and afraid. The One, however, knows no fear but is pure bliss.

Prayer and meditation necessarily proceed from our ordinary experience of being a subject confronting an objective world. In fact, we can tell their effectiveness by the degree to which they bridge the split between mind and matter, inside and outside. Successful meditation and prayer lead to the state of ecstatic unification in which subject and object stand revealed as the same eternal Being. This ecstatic self-transcendence must be realized not only in special moments of isolated contemplation but also in every moment of active life.

THE MIND MACHINE

The ordinary mind, being a machine, has but one function: It creates and then goes about attempting to solve problems! It enjoys this game and will continue to play it as long as you allow it to do so, throughout your entire life if it can. It is not concerned that you are suffering in many areas because of its games. You will come to understand through the meditation techniques that *you are not your ordinary mind* and that it has not nearly the importance which we attach to it.

—RICHARD HITTLEMAN

BRINGING THE MIND HOME

We are fragmented into so many different aspects. We don't know who we really are, or what aspects of ourselves we should identify with or believe in. So many contradictory voices, dictates, and feelings fight for control over our inner lives that we find ourselves scattered everywhere, in all directions, leaving nobody at home.

Meditation, then, is bringing the mind home. . . .

—SOGYAL RINPOCHE

THE MIND IS LIKE A BIRD

The mind is like a bird in a field, always pecking at and picking up something; what is important is that it should select wisely. All that the senses report is woven into something which tends either to destroy or to build up the mind, for the mind assimilates that upon which it dwells. . . . Hatred and fanaticism introduce qualities which coarsen the mind, impairing mental health; but selfless thoughts are pure, for they seek the well-being of all and unite the puny individual mind with the cosmic Mind, the mind of God, which rules alike the stars in their courses, the electrons in their orbits, and governs the emergence of the infinitely varied forms of life.

—HARI PRASAD SHASTRI

IMMORTAL MINDFULNESS

Mindfulness is the way of immortality—
Heedlessness the way of death.
The mindful will not die—
The heedless are perpetually dead.

—NAGARJUNA

THE ARROW OF
ONE-POINTED THOUGHT

The art of archery is to draw the arrow back on the bow as far as possible and then to release the arrow, sending it ahead with great force. Likewise, the mind should be drawn back to the source of thinking and, from there, released to bring the thought out in a forceful manner supplemented by the power of the Being. It will bring out a powerful thought that will succeed in the relative world, bring the infusion of the Being into outside activity, and make possible the state of cosmic consciousness.

—MAHARISHI MAHESH YOGI

THE POWER OF CONCENTRATION

Concentration is like a diamond, a brilliant focusing of our energy, intelligence, and sensitivity. When we concentrate fully, the light of our abilities shines forth in many colors, radiating through all that we do. Our energy gains a momentum and clarity that allows us to perform each task quickly and with ease, and we respond to the challenges work offers with pleasure and enthusiasm.

—TARTHANG TULKU

ONE-POINTED MIND

❧

When one learns to practice awareness and attention while doing even the simplest and most mundane acts of life, a great joy comes.

When water runs in scattered rivulets down the hillside, it hasn't much force behind it. But when it is dammed up and made to come through a narrow opening, its power is tremendous. Likewise, when sunlight is focused through a magnifying glass, that spot of light becomes powerful enough to burn.

So it is with our minds. A mind that wanders distracted, scattered, and inattentive has little power. But when its awareness is focused one-pointedly, it becomes so powerful that it can achieve anything. Such a mind gains spiritual power.

—BRAHMACHARINI NITYA

SURFING MEDITATION

When I'm out there on the ocean floating on my board, alone with the wind and the sky, I'm excruciatingly aware of how small and insignificant I am in comparison to the awesome power of the water. It would be presumptuous of me to say that I surf the waves—in fact, the waves surf me!

. . . Well, meditation is like surfing. If you push too hard and try to control your mind, you'll just end up feeling rigid and tight, and you'll keep wiping out as the result of your effort. But if you hang back and exert no effort at all, you won't have the focus or concentration necessary to hold your position as the waves of thought and emotion wash over you.

—STEPHAN BODIAN

DON'T TRY

Do not try. Trying and struggling to achieve a level of meditation always brings the opposite results.

—PANDIT USHARBUDH ARYA

WATCHING THE WATCHER

❧

Although we cannot really stop the process of I-making, we can disengage a certain part of ourselves from it and observe it. And when we learn to observe our thought patterns, we find that the conscious mind begins to change. A different sense of *ahamkara* comes into being—a different sense of "I" is watching, witnessing, dispassionately observing. Just as there are various levels of consciousness, so are there differing varieties of I-ness, and now we realize that in addition to the "I" who is being the typical me, there is another "I" who is watching it all.

—RUDOLPH M. BALLENTINE

MEDITATION IS DRILLING

୬

After a lot of sustained, systematic effort in meditation, we may finally succeed in breaking through the surface crust of consciousness. What lies below is the unconscious, which has many layers—strata on strata deposited by habits of thinking and acting, little by little, every day of our life. Drilling through these strata in meditation means overcoming limitations, all the obstacles created by self-will: the fierce, driving compulsion to have our own way, get what *we* want, stamp ourselves separate from the rest of life. The biggest leap in meditation comes when we run headlong and throw ourselves over the rim of all duality to land in the unitive state, where nothing is separate from the Lord. This state is *shanti*, perfect peace.

—EKNATH EASWARAN

WORSHIPPING IN THE TEMPLE OF THE BODY

Your body, and not any edifice built by human hands, is your living temple. Enter the inner silence, and worship there. Send rays of devotion in solemn procession up the aisle of the spine from your heart to the high altar in the forehead, the seat of superconscious ecstasy.

—J. DONALD WALTERS (SWAMI KRIYANANDA)

MEDITATION IS NO KALEIDOSCOPE

In meditation, you sometimes expect to experience foolish things—you want to see lights and colors. If you meditate with such ideas, you will never really meditate. Meditation means gently fathoming all the levels of yourself, one level after another. Be honest at least with yourself. Don't care what others say about practice—keep your mind focused on your goal.

—SWAMI RAMA

TRUTH ALONE

꒰

Meditation is the eye that sees the Truth, the heart that feels
the Truth and the soul that realizes the Truth.

—SRI CHINMOY

MEDITATION AND FREEDOM

꒰

Thought is not the way to the new. Only meditation opens
the door to that which is everlastingly new. Meditation is
not a trick of thought. It is the seeing of the futility of
thought and the ways of the intellect. Intellect and thought
are necessary in the operation of anything mechanical, but
the intellect is a fragmentary perception of the whole and
meditation is the seeing of the whole. Intellect can operate
only in the field of the known and that is why life becomes a
monotonous routine from which we try to escape through
revolts and revolutions—merely to fall back once again into
another field of the known. This change is no change at all
as it is the product of thought which is always old. Meditation is the flight from the known. There is only one freedom: it is, from the known. And beauty and love lie in this
freedom.

—JIDDU KRISHNAMURTI

A PORTABLE PARADISE

‿

"By the practice of meditation," the Master said, "you will find that you are carrying within your heart a portable paradise."
—PARAMAHANSA YOGANANDA

UNITING THOUGHT AND ACTION

‿

During the day do not do one thing while thinking about another. Thought and action must be unified—no thought be permitted without reference to action or intended action; and no action be performed without intention. By this practice all day long the mind and body are taught to act together, without any waste of physical or mental energy.
—ERNEST WOOD

MEDITATION AND LIFE

‿

Meditation must permeate life. Then problems of life will cease to distract the mind in meditation.
—PANDIT USHARBUDH ARYA

17

FREEDOM AND HAPPINESS

✑

According to Yoga philosophy, human life ordinarily revolves around the pursuit of three basic goals:

Artha—material comfort or security; prosperity
Kama—emotional and intellectual satisfaction, includ-
ing creativity
Dharma—justice and moral goodness

To these the Yoga masters have added the ideal of spiritual freedom (*moksha*), which is the same as Self-realization,
liberation, or enlightenment.

Statisticians tell us that over one billion people on our
planet are in survival mode. They do not have enough to eat
and have to make do with unsafe water. They are suffering
from malnutrition and have little or no room in their lives
for pleasurable activities. Their numbers are growing as the
world's population continues to spike.

Some three to four billion people have adequate food and
housing and live moderately comfortable lives. They still adhere to traditional standards of morality, but with increasing

affluence the consumer mentality creeps in, which erodes traditional values and behaviors.

Then there are the more than a billion citizens of developed countries who are comparatively well off and consume resources at an alarming rate. They could devote themselves to the spiritual goal of liberation but by and large are preoccupied with the pursuit of money (falling under the category of *artha*) and pleasure in all its numerous varieties, not least sexual pleasure. The problem is that no amount of pleasure can fulfill us. On the contrary, escalating pleasure deprives us of inner balance and obscures our spiritual nature. Despite the great affluence in the United States, for instance, mental health is at an all-time low.

While pleasure has its place in human life, it should not become an idol over which we obsess. Our potential as human beings is so much more magnificent than we tend to realize. Without a spiritual perspective, material wealth and the pursuit of "fun" or even the meticulous performance of our duty can become a veritable trap that deprives us of higher meaning, happiness, and freedom.

So long as we have not glimpsed our true identity, the Self or Spirit, we are enslaved to the mostly uninspected habit patterns of our own mind. Even though our democratic ideals include personal freedom, we seldom understand that freedom lies beyond the well-worn grooves of our brain. Thus we settle for the kind of freedom that allows us to merely assert our ego-bound will. Real freedom, however, is living out of the fullness and spontaneity of the Spirit, without guarantees but with unlimited courage and wisdom. Yoga makes our realization of such unparalleled freedom possible.

THE MANY FORMS OF FREEDOM

❧

Freedom is the one goal of all nature, sentient or insentient. And, consciously or unconsciously, everything is struggling towards that goal. The freedom which the saint seeks is very different from that which the robber seeks; the freedom loved by the saint leads him to the enjoyment of infinite, unspeakable bliss, while that on which the robber has set his heart only forges other bonds for his soul.

—SWAMI VIVEKANANDA

TOWARD INNER FREEDOM

❧

The whole trend of modern civilization is towards external freedom. Free expression of opinion, free association, freedom to establish one's personal relationships on one's own initiative, and freedom to pursue a vocation according to one's merits are essentially needed for making life fruitful and happy. But external freedom, in the last analysis, is egocentric, and should not miss its spiritual counterpart in internal freedom. Inner freedom consists in the conquest of lust, anger, greed, attachment, pride, and sloth. A happy blending of reason and love can alone bring about this freedom and give meaning to all forms of external freedom. The substance of all religions consists in the achievement of this inner freedom.

—SWAMI AVYAKTANANDA

ASLEEP, AWAKE, ENLIGHTENED

❧

Yoga classifies individuals as "sleeping," "awakened," or "enlightened." The "sleeping" man is not aware that he is using only a fraction of his great potential power. He plods his way through life in a conditioned hypnotic state as a prisoner of his ordinary mind and his five senses. He may be "successful" in all of the ways of the world. He may appear to be a man who is "happy" and "satisfied" in the ordinary sense of the words. And yet, if he has not been able to perceive what lies beyond his senses and has been unable to transcend his ordinary mind, the Yogi will say that this man is "asleep."

The "awakened" man realizes that he is not using his great reservoir of potential resources. He knows instinctively that there are powerful forces available to him if he can but learn how to utilize them. The "awakened" man is intuitively involved in attempting to contact and use his dormant power.

The "enlightened" man is the ultimate objective of Yoga practice. He has aroused his latent forces and controls them; he has transcended his ordinary mind and is able to integrate himself with the Universal Mind. As such, he is no longer affected by the fears, anxieties, and weaknesses of people still in bondage to these things.

—RICHARD HITTLEMAN

DISCOVERING THE HIGHER SELF

ॐ

The Self (*atman*) that is free from evil, free from old age and death, free from sorrow, hunger, and thirst, and whose desires and intentions are real—that you should seek out and know. He who has discovered that Self and has come to know it, obtains all the worlds and all desires.

—*CHANDOGYA-UPANISHAD*

SELF'S LUMINOSITY

ॐ

Take the sun: there are innumerable cloudlets in the sky. The rays of the sun are reflected through the clouds, and it is by virtue of the reflection of these rays that the clouds are perceptible. You cannot see them on a dark night. You see them by virtue of the sun's rays. Your Self is comparable to the sun and your mind is comparable to the little clouds.

—HARI PRASAD SHASTRI

INNER SUNRISE

When the sun rises, all the stars fade away in its brilliance. Similarly, when the sun of knowledge rises in the heart and a person experiences the essence of the Self, the universe of diversity with its countless beings and objects is dissolved for him. Duality perishes. The radiant sun of the Self blazes in his eyes. Its flame radiates through every pore of his body. As it flashes, his entire body is filled with the nectar of love.

—SWAMI MUKTANANDA

DAWNING OF THE INNER LIGHT

Sunrise in the sky of the heart is the most blessed sight.

—SWAMI NITYANANDA

FREEDOM

❧

When our inner nature is truly free, we find within ourselves a wealth of treasure: love, joy, and peace of mind. We can appreciate the beauty of life, taking each experience as it comes, opening our hearts to it and fully enjoying it. Realizing these qualities within ourselves is the greatest freedom that can be gained.

—Tarthang Tulku

HOME, SWEET HOME

❧

There is no home greater than Self-realization.

—Swami Jyotir Maya Nanda

SURRENDERING ALL

࿔

The ultimate attainment is already ours, but the experience of it comes to us only when we are in a state of complete surrender. In this case, "surrender" means the surrender of everything—every effort, desire, thought of attainment or, indeed, anything that represents the thought of any *other*—as we become centered, instead. The person who is able to do this becomes a fountain of consciousness.

—SWAMI CHETANANANDA

THE LUTE OF THE BODY

࿔

When life is purified and the lute of the body is perfectly tuned, the flow of the inner currents pervading the universe comes like a gust of wind and strikes the instrument. When there is a problem, or a difficulty or an obstacle, the man who is calm and unruffled and seriously in communion with his self is bound to come into contact with the universe. If the person is emotionally keen, a devotee or a lover, the current will take a visual form and lead the way. If he has a keen intelligence and has followed the path of knowledge, his mind will vibrate with perception and understanding. So the help he needs is pre-arranged.

—VIMALA THAKAR

SOUL'S MUSIC

Listen to the Music of the Soul
With the chords of your heart attuned
With the strings of your thoughts in unison
With the Divine Musician.

—SWAMI JYOTIR MAYA NANDA

INFINITY

I am now speaking and eating through so many mouths. I am the Soul of all individual souls. I have infinite mouths, infinite heads, infinite hands and feet. My pure form is spiritual. It is absolute Existence, Intelligence and Bliss condensed, as it were. It has neither birth nor death, neither sorrow, disease nor suffering. It is immortal and perfect. I see the indivisible Absolute Brahman within me as well as all around me. You are all like my own parts. The Infinite Brahman is manifesting Itself through so many human forms. Human bodies are like pillow-cases of different shapes and various colors, but the cotton wool of the internal Spirit is one.

—SRI RAMAKRISHNA

I AM NEITHER THIS NOR THAT

❧

I am neither the doer nor the enjoyer.
Actions have I none, now or then.
I have no body, nor am I bodiless.
How can there be "mine" and "not mine"?

I have no flaws like attachment,
Nor any suffering arising from embodiment.
Know me to be the singular Self,
As vast as space itself.

—*AVADHUTA-GITA*

THE FINAL ACCOUNT

❧

When the goal of life is attained, one achieves the reparation
of all wrongs, the healing of all wounds, the righting of all
failures, the sweetening of all sufferings, the relaxation of
all strivings, the harmonizing of all strife, the unraveling of
all enigmas, and the real and full meaning of all life—past,
present, and future.

—MEHER BABA

BIBLIOGRAPHIC REFERENCES

ANCIENT INVOCATION (PAGE V)
Brihad-Aranyaka-Upanishad (1.3.28). Translated from the original Sanskrit by Georg Feuerstein.

DEDICATION (PAGE VII)
Miguel de Unamuno

1. MIND—MAKER OF DESTINY

"YOU SHOULD WELCOME HEARTILY . . ." (PAGE 4)
Swami Muktananda, *Play of Consciousness: Chitshakt Vilas* (New York: Harper & Row, 1978), p. 245.

TO GROW OR NOT TO GROW (PAGE 5)
Swami Chetanananda, *The Breath of God* (Cambridge, Mass.: Rudra Press, 1988), p. 46.

BECOMING HUMAN (PAGE 6)
David Frawley, *Beyond the Mind* (Salt Lake City, Utah: Passage Press, 1992), p. 55.

LIFE IS PRECIOUS (PAGE 7)
Maharaj Charan Singh, *Spiritual Discourses,* 6th ed. (Punjab, India: Radha Soami Satsang Beas, 1991), pp. 33, 40.

YOU BECOME WHAT YOU THINK (PAGE 8)
Maitri-Upanishad (6.3.) Translated from the original Sanskrit by Georg Feuerstein.

BE CAREFUL WHAT YOU THINK (PAGE 8)
Sri Ananda Acharya, retold after Sri Ananda Acharya, *Yoga of Conquest* (Hoshiarpur, India: Vishveshvaranand Institute, 1971), p. 258.

MENTAL SUGGESTION (PAGE 9)
Swami Brahmananda, cited in *The Apostles of Shri Ramakrishna,* comp. and ed. by Swami Gambhirananda (Calcutta: Advaita Ashram, 1972), p. 114.

MENTAL POWER (PAGE 9)

Jnanadeva, *Jnaneshvari* (6.35). Paraphrase of the original Marathi text by Georg Feuerstein.

CONTROLLING THE BRAIN (PAGE 10)

Pundit Acharya, *Breath, Sleep, the Heart, and Life: The Revolutionary Health Yoga of Pundit Acharya* (Lower Lake, Calif.: The Dawn Horse Press, 1975), p. 11.

MIND CONTROL (PAGE 10)

Swami Rama, *Inner Paths* (Honesdale, Pa.: The Himalayan International Institute of Yoga Science and Philosophy, 1979), p. 15.

MENTAL PURITY (PAGE 11)

Swami Vijnanananda, cited in *The Apostles of Shri Ramakrishna,* comp. and ed. by Swami Gambhirananda (Calcutta: Advaita Ashram, 1972), p. 398.

THOUGHT AND ADDICTION (PAGE 11)

David Frawley, *Beyond the Mind* (Salt Lake City, Utah: Passage Press, 1992), p. 97.

CHOOSE A SUBLIME IDEAL (PAGE 12)

Omraam Mikhaël Aïvanhov, *Golden Rules for Everyday Life* (Fréjus, France: Editions Prosveta, 1990), pp. 17–18.

MAKING LIFE MEANINGFUL (PAGE 12)

Lama Anagarika Govinda, *Foundations of Tibetan Mysticism* (London: Rider, 1969), p. 277.

RIGHT UNDERSTANDING (PAGE 13)

Nagarjuna, *The Precious Garland and The Song of the Four Mindfulnesses,* trans. and ed. by Jeffrey Hopkins and Lati Rimpoche with Anne Klein (London: George Allen and Unwin Ltd., 1975), p. 35 (verses 121–22).

RIGHT VIEW (PAGE 14)

Ron Leifer, *The Happiness Project* (Ithaca, N.Y.: Snow Lion Publications, 1997), p. 63.

FROM IGNORANCE TO KNOWLEDGE (PAGE 15)

Sri Aurobindo, *A Practical Guide to Integral Yoga*, 7th ed. (Pondicherry, India: Sri Aurobindo Ashram, 1976), p. 208.

THE MILK OF WISDOM (PAGE 15)

Brahma-Bindu-Upanishad (20). Translated from the original Sanskrit by Georg Feuerstein.

TWO KINDS OF DOUBT (PAGE 16)

Paramahansa Yogananda, *Sayings of Yogananda* (Los Angeles: Self-Realization Fellowship, 1968), p. 59.

THE LIMITS OF REASON (PAGE 16)

Swami Sivananda Saraswati, *Practice of Yoga*, 4th ed. (Sivanandanagar, India: The Divine Life Society, 1970), p. 439.

MENTAL CLOUDS (PAGE 17)

Swami Sivananda Radha, *Kundalini Yoga for the West* (Spokane, Wash.: Timeless Books, 1978), p.177.

FAITH (PAGE 17)

Swami Satyasangananda Saraswati, *Light on the Guru and Disciple Relationship* (Bihar, India: Bihar School of Yoga, 1984), p. 191.

THE MIND MUST BE AWAKENED (PAGE 18)

Maharaj Charan Singh, *Spiritual Discourses*, 6th ed. (Punjab, India: Radha Soami Satsang Beas, 1991), p. 70.

FOOLS AND SAGES (PAGE 18)

Vardhamana Mahavira, *Akaranga-Sutra* (3.1.1). Translated from the original Prakrit by Georg Feuerstein.

THE SECRET OF PROPER DISCERNMENT (PAGE 19)

Selvarajan Yesudian, *A Yoga Miscellany: A Collection of Class Lectures and Explanatory Texts for Students of Yoga* (London: George Allen & Unwin, 1963), p. 80.

PERFECT MIND, PERFECT HEART (PAGE 20)

"Mahatma" M.K. Gandhi, *The Mind of Mahatma Gandhi*, ed. by R. K. Prabhu and U. R. Rao (Ahmedabad, India: Navajivan Publishing House, 1967), pp. 82–83.

THE HIGHEST HELP (PAGE 20)

Swami Vivekananda, *Karma-Yoga and Bhakti-Yoga* (New York: Ramakrishna-Vivekananda Center, 1982), p. 32.

2. THE QUEST

IN SEARCH OF LIGHT (PAGE 23)
Sri Ananda Acharya, *Yoga of Conquest* (Hoshiarpur, India: Vishvesh-varanand Institute, 1971), p. 170.

OVERCOMING LIMITATIONS (PAGE 23)
Vimala Thakar, *Life as Yoga* (Delhi, India: Motilal Banarsidass, 1977), p. 190.

DIGGING UP THE HIDDEN TREASURE (PAGE 24)
Swami Muktananda, *Secret of the Siddhas,* 3rd printing (South Fallsburg, N.Y.: SYDA Foundation, 1983), p. 60.

DISCOVERING MIRACLES WITHIN (PAGE 24)
Swami Chidvilasananda, *The Yoga of Discipline* (South Fallsburg, N.Y.: SYDA Foundation, 1996), p. 138.

LEARNING THE GREAT LESSON (PAGE 25)
Hari Prasad Shastri, *Self-Knowledge* (London: Shanti Sadan, Winter 1997), p. 8.

THE QUEST (PAGE 25)
Paul Brunton, *The Notebooks of Paul Brunton,* vol. 2, *The Quest* (Burdett, N.Y.: Larson Publications, 1986), pp. 4–8.

ASKING THE RIGHT QUESTIONS (PAGE 26)
Shivapuri Baba, Renu Lal Singh, *Right Life: Teachings of Shivapuri Baba* (Moorcote, England: Coombe Springs Press, 1984), p. 25.

LONGING FOR LIBERATION (PAGE 26)
Sri Ananda Acharya, *Yoga of Conquest* (Hoshiarpur, India: Vishvesh-varanand Institute, 1971), pp. 90–91.

THE BIG QUESTION (PAGE 27)
David Frawley, *Beyond the Mind* (Salt Lake City, Utah: Passage Press, 1992), p. 121.

YEARNING TO GROW (PAGE 27)
Swami Chetanananda, *The Breath of God* (Cambridge, Mass.: Rudra Press, 1973), p. 49.

ASPIRING TO WISDOM'S LIGHT (PAGE 28)
Hari Prasad Shastri, *Self-Knowledge* (London: Shanti Sadan, Summer 1995), p. 84.

3. THE TEACHER—GUIDING LIGHT

A HELPING HAND FROM HEAVEN (PAGE 32)
Paul Brunton, *The Notebooks of Paul Brunton,* vol. 2, *The Quest* (Burdett, N.Y.: Larson Publications, 1986), pp. 222–33.

THE TEACHER IS AN INSTRUMENT (PAGE 32)
Munishree Chitrabhanu, cited in Swami Rama, *Inner Paths* (Honesdale, Pa.: The Himalayan International Institute of Yoga Science and Philosophy, 1979), p. 52.

THE DUAL PURPOSE OF THE TEACHER (PAGE 33)
Swami Chetanananda, *The Breath of God* (Cambridge, Mass.: Rudra Press, 1973), p. 40.

THE RIGHT APPROACH TO TEACHERS (PAGE 34)
David Frawley, "Missing the Mark: Western Illusions about Gurus," *Yoga International,* January/February 1992, p. 19.

TEACH YOURSELF (PAGE 34)
Swami Vivekananda, *Karma-Yoga and Bhakti-Yoga* (New York: Ramakrishna-Vivekananda Center, 1982), p. 81.

INNER *GURU,* OUTER *GURU* (PAGE 35)
Swami Satyasangananda Saraswati, *Light on the Guru and Disciple Relationship,* 1st enlarged Indian edition (Munger, India: Bihar School of Yoga, 1984), pp. 5, 7, 203.

4. FIRST STEPS ON THE PATH

A COLORFUL PERSONALITY (PAGE 38)
Pandit Usharbudh Arya, *Superconscious Meditation* (Honesdale, Pa.: Himalayan International Institute of Yoga Science and Philosophy, 1974 and 1978), pp. 33, 21.

BEYOND APPEARANCE (PAGE 39)
Swami Chetanananda, *Dynamic Stillness: Part Two: The Practice of Trika Yoga* (Cambridge, Mass.: Rudra Press, 1990), p. 39.

THE OTHER SIDE OF COMFORT (PAGE 39)
Swami Avyaktananda, *Letters to a Truth-Seeker* (London: The Vedanta Movement, 1943), p. 53.

THE TWO KEYS OF LIFE (PAGE 40)
Sri Ananda Acharya, *Yoga of Conquest* (Hoshiarpur, India: Vishvesh-varanand Institute, 1971), p. 229.

SHIFTING ONE'S OUTLOOK (PAGE 43)
Swami Viprananda, "A Stone in Water," *Yoga International,* November/December 1994, p. 18.

KNOWING WHAT YOU DON'T WANT (PAGE 43)
Swami Chetanananda, *Dynamic Stillness: Part Two: The Practice of Trika Yoga* (Cambridge, Mass.: Rudra Press, 1990), p. 16.

THE EIGHTFOLD PATH (PAGE 44)
Paramahansa Yogananda, "A World Without Boundaries," in Paramahansa Yogananda et al., *A World in Transition: Finding Spiritual Security in Times of Change* (Los Angeles: Self-Realization Fellowship, 1999), pp. 159–60.

DON'T JUST SIT THERE (PAGE 45)
Omraam Mikhaël Aïvanhov, *The Seeds of Happiness* (Fréjus, France: Prosveta S.A., 1992), pp. 3–4.

A SINGLE PURPOSE (PAGE 46)
Sri Ananda Acharya, *Yoga of Conquest* (Hoshiarpur, India: Vishvesh-varanand Institute, 1971), p. 71.

STOP NIBBLING (PAGE 46)
Swami Vivekananda, *Raja Yoga* (Mayavati, India: Advaita Ashrama, 1962), p. 85.

SINCERE EFFORT (PAGE 47)
Swami Rama, *Inspired Thoughts of Swami Rama* (Honesdale, Pa.: The Himalayan International Institute of Yoga Science and Philosophy of the U.S.A., 1983), p. 97.

THE PRINCIPLE CONDITION FOR SUCCESS (PAGE 47)
Sri Aurobindo, *A Practical Guide to Integral Yoga,* 7th ed. (Pondicherry, India: Sri Aurobindo Ashram, 1976), p. 63.

CONSISTENT CHEERFUL EFFORT (PAGE 48)
Rohit Mehta, *Yoga: The Art of Integration: A Commentary on the Yoga Sutras of Patanjali* (Adyar, Madras, India: The Theosophical Publishing House, 1975), pp. 27–28.

TRANSFORM YOUR MIND THROUGH STUDY (PAGE 49)
Swami Chidananda, *The Philosophy, Psychology and Practice of Yoga* (Distr. Tehri Garhwal, India: The Divine Life Society, 1984), p. 70.

SELF-OBSERVATION (PAGE 49)
Swami Rama, *The Art of Joyful Living* (Honesdale, Pa: Himalayan International Institute of Yoga Science and Philosophy, 1989), p. 111.

THE POISON OF FORCED DISCIPLINE (PAGE 50)
Maharaj Charan Singh, *Spiritual Discourses*, 6th ed. (Punjab, India: Radha Soami Satsang Beas, 1991), p. 93.

UPLIFT YOURSELF BY THE SELF (PAGE 50)
Bhagavad-Gita (6.5). Translated from the original Sanskrit by Georg Feuerstein. The Sanskrit language has no capital letters, and so the word *atman* can mean both the lower self and the higher Self. It is up to the translator to offer the most plausible interpretation.

5. CHALLENGING THE EGO

THE TRUTH ABOUT US (PAGE 53)
Alan Watts, *Om: Creative Meditations from Alan Watts*, ed. and adpt. by Judith Johnstone (Berkeley, Calif.: Celestial Arts, 1980), p. 90.

IMPRISONED BY THE EGO (PAGE 53)
Paul Brunton, *The Notebooks of Paul Brunton,* vol. 6, *From Birth to Rebirth* (Burdett, New York: Larson Publications, 1987), part 1, p. 70.

THE EGO IS NOT AN ENTITY (PAGE 54)
Bubba Free John (Adi Da), *The Paradox of Instruction* (San Francisco: Dawn Horse Press, 1977), p. 103.

THE EGO AS CONTRACTION (PAGE 54)
Swami Chetanananda, *Dynamic Stillness: Part Two: The Practice of Trika Yoga* (Cambridge, Mass.: Rudra Press, 1990), p. 31.

THE ONLY FOE (PAGE 55)
Swami Premananda, cited in *The Apostles of Shri Ramakrishna,* comp. and ed. by Swami Gambhirananda (Calcutta: Advaita Ashram, 1972), p. 144.

WILLPOWER OVER EGO POWER (PAGE 55)
Pandit Rajmani Tigunait, Inner Quest column, *Yoga International,* March/April 1992, p. 47.

THE ULTIMATE SHAPE-SHIFTER (PAGE 56)
Swami Niranjanananda Saraswati, *Yoga Sadhana Panorama,* vol. 1 (Munger, India: Bihar School of Yoga, 1995), p. 176.

THE EGO IS A HABIT (PAGE 56)
Jean Klein, *Neither This Nor That I Am* (London and Dulverton, England: Watkins Publishing, 1981), p. 105.

WHITTLING AWAY THE EGO (PAGE 57)
Swami Gitananda Giri, *Frankly Speaking* (Chinnamudaliarchavady, India: Satya Press, 1997), pp. 112–13.

SELF-CONTROL (PAGE 57)
Uttaradhyayana-Sutra (1.15). Translated from the original Prakrit by Georg Feuerstein. This *Sutra* belongs to the Jaina canon.

6. THE GOOD LIFE

THE MAGIC OF VIRTUE (PAGE 60)
Swami Jyotirmayananda, *The Art of Positive Feeling* (South Miami, Fla.: Yoga Research Foundation, 1997), p. 50.

SPIRITUAL LIFE AND MORALS (PAGE 60)
"Mahatma" M. K. Gandhi, *The Mind of Mahatma Gandhi,* ed. by R. K. Prabhu and U. R. Rao (Ahmedabad, India: Navajivan Publishing House, 1967), p. 101.

SPIRITUAL RECIPROCITY (PAGE 61)
Maharishi Mahesh Yogi, *Transcendental Meditation* (New York: The New American Library, 1963), p. 89.

THE JOY OF SERVICE (PAGE 61)
Pandit Rajmani Tigunait, *Yoga on War and Peace* (Honesdale, Pa.: The Himalayan International Institute of Yoga Science and Philosophy of the U.S.A., 1991), p. 104.

JOYOUS ACTION (PAGE 62)
Thynn Thynn, *Living Meditation, Living Insight: The Path of Mindfulness in Daily Life* (Sebastopol, Calif.: Sae Taw Win II Dhamma Center, 1998), p. 92.

THE YOGA OF SELF-TRANSCENDING ACTION (PAGE 62)
Bhagavad-Gita (2.47–48). Translated from the original Sanskrit by Georg Feuerstein.

EGO-TRANSCENDING ACTION (PAGE 63)
Milarepa, *The Hundred Thousand Songs of Milarepa,* trans. by Garma C. C. Change, abridged ed. (New York: Harper & Row, 1962), p. 17.

COMPETING *WITH* OTHERS (PAGE 63)
Tarthang Tulku, *Skillful Means* (Berkeley, Calif.: Dharma Publishing, 1978), pp. 89–90.

WORK AND WORSHIP (PAGE 64)
Swami Brahmananda, cited in *The Apostles of Shri Ramakrishna,* comp. and ed. by Swami Gambhirananda (Calcutta: Advaita Ashram, 1972), pp. 115–16.

FLOWER POWER (PAGE 64)
Swami Karmananda Saraswati, *Yogic Management of Common Diseases* (Bihar, India: Bihar School of Yoga, 1983), p. 87.

CHOOSE YOUR FRIENDS WISELY (PAGE 65)
Sri Ananda Acharya, *Yoga of Conquest* (Hoshiarpur, India: Vishveshvaranand Institute, 1971), pp. 65, 88.

TRUTH REIGNS SUPREME (PAGE 65)
Mahanirvana-Tantra (4.75). Translated from the original Sanskrit by Georg Feuerstein.

UNTRUTH UNDERMINES ALL (PAGE 66)
Vimala Thakar, *Life as Yoga* (Delhi, India: Motilal Banarsidass, 1977), p. 259.

HUMILITY AND GRATITUDE (PAGE 66)
Swami Sivananda Radha, *Kundalini Yoga for the West* (Spokane, Wash.: Timeless Books, 1978), p. 191.

HUMILITY THROUGH SELF-UNDERSTANDING (PAGE 67)
Tarthang Tulku, *Skillful Means* (Berkeley, Calif.: Dharma Publishing, 1978), pp. 124–25.

PATIENCE (PAGE 68)
Eknath Easwaran, *Thousand Names of Vishnu* (Petaluma, Calif.: Nilgiri Press, 1987), pp. 57, 59.

SICKENING SPEED (PAGE 69)
Meher Baba, Eknath Easwaran, *Meditation: A Simple Eight-Point Program for Translating Spiritual Ideals into Daily Life* (Tomales, Calif.: Nilgiri Press, 1978, 1991), p. 31.

LUMINOUS SLEEP (PAGE 69)
Omraam Mikhaël Aïvanhov, *Looking into the Invisible: Intuition, Clairvoyance, Dreams* (Fréjus, France: Prosveta S.A., 1989), p. 160.

NOCTURNAL YOGI (PAGE 70)
Paramahansa Yogananda, *Autobiography of a Yogi* (Los Angeles: Self-Realization Fellowship, 1987), p. 281.

7. TAMING THE EMOTIONS

FOLLOW YOUR HEART (PAGE 74)
Swami Akhandananda, cited in *The Apostles of Shri Ramakrishna*, comp. and ed. by Swami Gambhirananda (Calcutta: Advaita Ashram, 1972), p. 364.

FEELINGS AND DESTINY (PAGE 74)
Sri Ananda Acharya, *Yoga of Conquest* (Hoshiarpur, India: Vishveshvaranand Institute, 1971), pp. 67–68.

EMOTIONAL PURIFICATION (PAGE 74)
Pandit Usharbudh Arya, *Superconscious Meditation* (Honesdale, Pa.: Himalayan International Institute of Yoga Science and Philosophy, 1974, 1978), p. 81.

TAMED EMOTIONS (PAGE 75)
Swami Sivananda Radha, *Mantras: Words of Power* (Porthill, Idaho: Timeless, 1980), p. 23.

LIBERATING EMOTION (PAGE 76)
Tenzin Wangyal Rinpoche, *The Tibetan Yogas of Dream and Sleep* (Ithaca, N.Y.: Snow Lion Publications, 1998), p. 30.

EMOTIONAL CHAIN REACTION (PAGE 77)
Vardhamana Mahavira, *Acaranga-Sutra* (4.4.4). Translated from the original Prakrit by Georg Feuerstein.

ENSNARED CONSCIOUSNESS (PAGE 77)
Yoga-Vasishtha (5.34.104). Translated from the original Sanskrit by Georg Feuerstein.

JOY BEYOND FUN (PAGE 78)
Eknath Easwaran, *Thousand Names of Vishnu* (Petaluma, Calif.: Nilgiri Press, 1987), p. 135.

MIND'S WEB (PAGE 78)
Dhammapada (18.251). Translated from the original Pali by Georg Feuerstein.

ADAMANTINE DESIRE (PAGE 79)
Swami Jyotirmayananda, *The Art of Positive Feeling* (South Miami, Fla.: Yoga Research Foundation, 1997), p. 25.

THE TRUTH ABOUT DESIRE (PAGE 79)
Paul Brunton, *Essays on the Quest* (York Beach, Maine: Samuel Weiser, 1984), p. 166.

FACING THE TIGER (PAGE 80)
Vimala Thaker, *Life as Yoga* (Delhi, India: Motilal Banarsidass, 1977), pp. 125–26.

CONQUERING FEAR (PAGE 81)
Swami Shri Kripalvanandji, *Pilgrimage of Love, Book II* (Lenox, Mass.: Kripalu Publications, 1982), pp. 243–44.

HARNESSING THE ENERGY OF ANGER (PAGE 82)
Swami Chetanananda, *The Breath of God* (Cambridge, Mass.: Rudra Press, 1973), p. 186.

MELTING AWAY ANGER (PAGE 83)
Thynn Thynn, *Living Meditation, Living Insight: The Path of Mindfulness in Daily Life* (Sebastopol, Calif.: Sae Taw Win II Dhamma Center, 1998), p. 27.

OVERCOMING NEGATIVITY THROUGH WITNESSING (PAGE 83)
Aruna Bhargava, "The Secret of Happiness," *Yoga International*, September/October 1991, p. 12.

THE PURSUIT OF POWER (PAGE 84)
David Frawley, *Beyond the Mind* (Salt Lake City, Utah: Passage Press, 1992), p. 141.

OVERCOMING ANGER (PAGES 84–85)
Geshe Jampa Gyatso, *Everlasting Rain of Nectar: Purification Practice in Tibetan Buddhism* (Boston: Wisdom Publications, New York and Oxford: Oxford University Press, 1996), p. 89.

AMBITION (PAGE 85)
Pandit Usharbudh Arya, *Superconscious Meditation* (Honesdale, Pa.:

Himalayan International Institute of Yoga Science and Philosophy, 1974, 1978), p. 97.

OVERCOMING JEALOUSY (PAGE 86)
Swami Jyotirmayananda, *The Art of Positive Feeling* (South Miami, Fla.: Yoga Research Foundation, 1997), p. 167.

CRITICISM IS ALWAYS CONSTRUCTIVE (PAGE 86)
Satguru Sivaya Subramaniyaswami, "Critical Collection," *Hinduism Today*, December 1996, p. 8.

CORRECT FAULT-FINDING (PAGE 87)
Atisha, *Vimala-Ratna-Lekha* (7a), cited in *Atisha and Buddhism in Tibet,* comp. and trans. by Dobbom Tulku and Glenn H. Mullin (New Delhi: Tibet House, 1983), p. 35.

DON'T JUDGE OTHERS (PAGE 87)
Hari Prasad Shastri, *Self-Knowledge* (London: Shanti Sadan, Summer 1992), p. 66.

HEALING WORDS (PAGE 88)
Omraam Mikhaël Aïvanhov, *Golden Rules for Everyday Life* (Fréjus, France: Prosveta, 1990), p. 73.

PEACE OVERCOMES ENMITY (PAGE 88)
The Dalai Lama, *Beyond Dogma: Dialogues & Discourses* (Berkeley, Calif.: North Atlantic Books, 1996), p. 88.

THE FRUIT OF NONVIOLENCE (PAGE 89)
Alice Christensen, *Yoga of the Heart* (New York: Daybreak Books, 1998), p. 62.

GENTLENESS (PAGE 89)
Swami Rama, *Inspired Thoughts of Swami Rama* (Honesdale, Pa.: The Himalayan International Institute of Yoga Science and Philosophy of the U.S.A., 1983), p. 22.

CHEERFULNESS (PAGE 90)
Pandit Rajmani Tigunait, *Yoga on War and Peace* (Honesdale, Pa.: The Himalayan International Institute of Yoga Science and Philosophy of the U.S.A., 1991), p. 108.

PILGRIMAGE TO COMPASSION (PAGE 90)
Swami Shri Kripalvanandji, *Pilgrimage of Love, Book II* (Lenox, Mass.: Kripalu Publications, 1982), p. 343.

INFINITE COMPASSION (PAGE 91)
Shantideva, *Bodhicaryavatara* (10:55). Translated from the original Sanskrit by Georg Feuerstein.

HAPPINESS FOR EVERYONE (PAGE 91)
The Dalai Lama, *Beyond Dogma: Dialogues & Discourses* (Berkeley, Calif.: North Atlantic Books, 1996), p. 5.

8. MASTERING THE MATERIAL WORLD

TRUE WEALTH (PAGE 94)
Omraam Mikhaël Aïvanhov, *Golden Rules for Everyday Life* (Fréjus, France: Prosveta, 1990), p. 46.

RENUNCIATION BEYOND CONTROL (PAGE 94)
David Frawley, *Beyond the Mind* (Salt Lake City, Utah: Passage Press, 1992), p. 154.

TRUE DETACHMENT (PAGE 95)
Swami Jyotirmayananda, *The Art of Positive Thinking* (South Miami, Fla.: Yoga Research Foundation, 1988), pp. 94–95.

CULTIVATE SIMPLICITY (PAGE 95)
Maggie Kramm, "Cultivating Simplicity," *Yoga International,* December/January 1997, p. 27.

NONATTACHMENT IS LIBERATING (PAGE 96)
Kula-Arnava-Tantra (1.55). Translated from the original Sanskrit by Georg Feuerstein.

MONEY (PAGE 96)
Sri Aurobindo, *A Practical Guide to Integral Yoga,* 7th ed. (Pondicherry, India: Sri Aurobindo Ashram, 1976), p. 262.

MONEY WORSHIP (PAGE 97)
Eknath Easwaran, *Thousand Names of Vishnu* (Petaluma, Calif.: Nilgiri Press, 1987), p. 129.

THE SOURCE OF ALL WEALTH (PAGE 98)
Baba Prakashananda, retold from Titus Foster, *Agaram Bagaram Baba: Life, Teachings, and Parables—A Spiritual Biography of Baba Prakashananda* (Berkeley, Calif.: North Atlantic Books, and Patagonia, Ariz.: Essene Vision Books, 1999), p. 140.

9. FOOD FOR THOUGHT

EAT WITH AWARENESS (PAGE 101)
Carrie Angus, "Food for the Wise," *Yoga International,* March/April 1996, p. 27.

FOR THE YOGI COOK (PAGE 102)
Jack Santa Maria, *Anna Yoga: The Yoga of Food* (London: Rider and Company, 1978), p. 107.

NUTRITIONAL YOGA (PAGE 103)
Omraam Mikhaël Aïvanhov, *Golden Rules for Everyday Life* (Fréjus, France: Prosveta, 1990), p. 20.

FOOD AND MENTAL HARMONY (PAGE 103)
Indra Devi, *Yoga for Americans* (Englewood Cliffs, N.J.: Prentice-Hall, 1959), pp. 83–84.

THE DISCIPLINE OF EATING (PAGE 104)
Swami Chidvilasananda, *The Yoga of Discipline* (South Fallsburg, N.Y.: SYDA Foundation, 1996), p. 138.

FOOD AS MEDICINE (PAGE 104)
Nagarjuna, cited in The Venerable Rendawa, Zhon-Nu Lo-Dro, *Nagarjuna's Letter*, trans. by Geshe Lobsang Tharching and Artemus B. Engle (Dharamsala, India: Library of Tibetan Works & Archives, 1979), p. 71.

SENSUAL FASTING (PAGE 105)
Jack Santa Maria, *Anna Yoga: The Yoga of Food* (London: Rider and Company, 1978), p. 101.

DELIGHT IN THE SIMPLE THINGS (PAGE 105)
Vijnana-Bhairava (72). Translated from the original Sanskrit by Georg Feuerstein.

10. MAKING PROGRESS

WE ARE OUR OWN REMEDY (PAGE 108)
Ron Leifer, *The Happiness Project* (Ithaca, N.Y.: Snow Lion Publications, 1997), p. 17.

ON BEING SPIRITUAL (PAGE 108)
Roy Eugene Davis, *The Eternal Way: The Inner Meaning of the Bhagavad Gita* (Lakemont, Ga.: CSA Press, Publishers, 1996), p. 292.

BE YOUR OWN BEST FRIEND (PAGE 109)

Munishree Chitrabhanu, cited in Swami Rama, *Inner Paths* (Honesdale, Pa.: The Himalayan International Institute of Yoga Science and Philosophy, 1979), p. 61.

GROWING MORE AND MORE AWARE (PAGE 109)

Swami Sivananda Radha, *Kundalini Yoga for the West* (Spokane, Wash.: Timeless Books, 1978), p. 10.

KNOW YOUR TEMPERAMENT (PAGE 110)

Bernard Bouanchaud, *The Essence of Yoga: Reflections on the* Yoga Sutras *of Patanjali* (Portland, Ore.: Rudra Press, 1997), p. 31.

GOOD VIBRATIONS FROM SELF-DISCIPLINE (PAGE 111)

Pandit Usharbudh Arya, *Superconscious Meditation* (Honesdale, Pa.: Himalayan International Institute of Yoga Science and Philosophy, 1974, 1978), p. 116.

REINING IN THE SENSES (PAGE 111)

Eknath Easwaran, *Thousand Names of Vishnu* (Petaluma, Calif.: Nilgiri Press, 1987), p. 102.

ATTENTIVENESS (PAGE 112)

Sri Ananda Acharya, *Yoga of Conquest* (Hoshiarpur, India: Vishveshvaranand Institute, 1971), p. 92.

CENTERING (PAGE 112)

Sri Daya Mata, cited in Linda Johnsen, "Only Love: A Conversation with Sri Daya Mata," *Yoga International,* July/August 1992, p. 24.

NOBILITY (PAGE 112)

Sri Ananda Acharya, *Yoga of Conquest* (Hoshiarpur, India: Vishveshvaranand Institute, 1971), p. 228.

HOW TO BECOME TRULY BEAUTIFUL (PAGE 113)

Swami Jyotir Maya Nanda, *Yoga Quotations from the Wisdom of Swami Jyotir Maya Nanda,* ed. by Swami Lalitananda (Miami, Fla.: International Yoga Society, 1975), p. 21.

TIME IS PRECIOUS (PAGE 113)

Tarthang Tulku, *Skillful Means* (Berkeley, Calif.: Dharma Publishing, 1978), p. 35.

CONQUERING COMPLACENCY (PAGE 114)
Swami Jyotirmayananda, *The Art of Positive Thinking* (South Miami, Fla.: Yoga Research Foundation, 1988), p. 31.

IDLENESS (PAGE 114)
Swami Rama, *The Art of Joyful Living* (Honesdale, Pa.: Himalayan International Institute of Yoga Science and Philosophy, 1989), p. 136.

ENTHUSIASM (PAGE 115)
Swami Chidvilasananda, *Enthusiasm* (South Fallsburg, N.Y.: SYDA Foundation, 1997), p. 27.

CONTROLLING NERVOUS HABITS (PAGE 115)
Richard Hittleman, *Guide to Yoga Meditation* (New York: Bantam Books, 1969), pp. 63–64.

ENERGY LEAKAGE (PAGE 116)
Swami Sivananda Saraswati, *Practice of Yoga,* rev. 4th ed. (Dist. Tehri-Garhwal, India: The Divine Life Society, 1970), p. 73.

THE TRAFFIC BODHISATTVA (PAGE 116)
Thich Nhat Hanh, "Driving," *Breath Sweeps Mind: A First Guide to Meditation Practice,* ed. by Jean Smith (New York: Riverhead Books, 1998), p. 178.

DYNAMIC TRANQUILITY (PAGE 117)
Rudolph M. Ballentine, *The Theory and Practice of Meditation* (Honesdale, Pa.: The Himalayan International Institute of Yoga Science and Philosophy of the U.S.A., 1986), p. 88.

HOW IMPERFECTIONS VANISH (PAGE 118)
Saraha, *Royal Dohas,* verses 10–11. Paraphrase of the Tibetan original by Georg Feuerstein.

SYMMETRY (PAGE 118)
B.K.S. Iyengar, *Iyengar: His Life and His Work* (Porthill, Idaho: Timeless Books, 1987), p. 499.

11. DEALING WITH DIFFICULTIES

DIFFICULTIES ARE POTTING SOIL (PAGE 121)
Omraam Mikhaël Aïvanhov, *Cosmic Balance* (Fréjus, France: Prosveta, 1996), p. 120.

THE INNER OBSTACLE RACE (PAGE 121)
Swami Satchidananda, *The Yoga Sutras of Patanjali* (Yogaville, Va.: Integral Yoga Publications, 1997), p. 51.

PAIN AS TEACHER (PAGE 122)
Swami Chetanananda, *Dynamic Stillness: Part Two: The Practice of Trika Yoga* (Cambridge, Mass.: Rudra Press, 1990), p. 75.

GROWING PAINS (PAGE 122)
Brother Anandamoy, cited in Margaret Wolff, "The Psychology of the Soul: An Inerview with Brother Anandamoy," *Yoga International*, November/December 1994, p. 33.

LIVING IN THE WORLD (PAGE 123)
Swami Satchidananda, cited in Deborah Willoughby, "Becoming a Seeker: An Interview with Swami Satchidananda," *Yoga International*, November/December 1992, p. 31.

PROTECT YOURSELF WITH LIGHT (PAGE 124)
Omraam Mikhaël Aïvanhov, *Golden Rules for Everyday Life* (Fréjus, France: Prosveta, 1990), p. 91.

THE GRACE OF DESPAIR (PAGE 125)
Pandit Usharbudh Arya. *God* (Honesdale, Pa.: The Himalayan International Institute of Yoga Science and Philosophy, 1979), pp. 45–46.

TWOFOLD GRACE (PAGE 125)
Swami Prabhavananda, "Grace and Self-Effort: Catching the Wind," *Yoga International*, May/June 1996, p. 65.

THE DEEPS OF THE PATH (PAGE 126)
Charles Breaux, *Journey into Consciousness: The Chakras, Tantra and Jungian Psychology* (York Beach, Maine: Nicolas-Hays, 1989), p. xvii.

PASSING THROUGH DRY SPELLS (PAGES 126–27)
Jack Santa Maria, *Anna Yoga: The Yoga of Food* (London: Rider and Company, 1978), pp. 57–58

REBALANCING WITH YOGA (PAGE 128)
Swami Karmananda Saraswati, *Yogic Management of Common Diseases* (Bihar, India: Bihar School of Yoga, 1983), unnumbered front page.

DEALING WITH DIFFICULTIES ON THE PATH (PAGES 128–29)
Swami Gitananda Giri, *Frankly Speaking* (Chinnamudaliarchavady, India: Satya Press, 1997), pp. 16–17.

FINDING RELIEF (PAGE 130)
Shri Yogendra, *Facts about Yoga* (Santa Cruz, Bombay, India: The Yoga Institute, 1975), p. 166.

DON'T WORRY, BE HAPPY (PAGE 130)
Swami Jyotirmayananda, *The Art of Positive Thinking* (South Miami, Fla.: Yoga Research Foundation, 1988), pp. 58–59.

USING EMOTIONAL ENERGY (PAGE 131)
Tarthang Tulku, *Skillful Means* (Berkeley, Calif.: Dharma Publishing, 1978), pp. 55–56.

NO PROBLEM (PAGE 132)
Swami Chetanananda, *Dynamic Stillness: Part Two: The Practice of Trika Yoga* (Cambridge, Mass.: Rudra Press, 1990), p. 53.

12. EMBODYING THE SPIRIT

BE FRIENDLY TOWARD YOUR BODY (PAGE 135)
Swami Karmananda Saraswati, *Yogic Management of Common Diseases* (Bihar, India: Bihar School of Yoga, 1983), p. 38.

IN YOUR OWN IMAGE (PAGE 135)
Charles Breaux, *Journey into Consciousness: The Chakras, Tantra and Jungian Psychology* (York Beach, Maine: Nicolas-Hays, 1989), p. 43.

YOU ARE NOT THE BODY (PAGE 136)
Swami Chetanananda, *Dynamic Stillness: Part Two: The Practice of Trika Yoga* (Cambridge, Mass.: Rudra Press, 1990), p. 35.

THE BODY IS AN AIRPLANE (PAGE 137)
Rammurti S. Mishra, *The Textbook of Yoga Psychology* (London: The Lyrebird Press Ltd., 1972), pp. 93–94.

YOUR BODY IS YOUR CHILD (PAGE 138)
Richard Hittleman, *Guide to Yoga Meditation* (New York: Bantam Books, 1969), p. 26.

MY BODY, MY TEACHER (PAGE 138)
Krishna, cited in the *Uddhava-Gita* (4.25). Translated from the original Sanskrit by Georg Feuerstein.

Feeling the Whole Body (page 139)
Tenzin Wangyal Rinpoche, *The Tibetan Yogas of Dream and Sleep* (Ithaca, N.Y.: Snow Lion Publications, 1998), p. 135.

The Body's Truth (page 140)
Judith Lasater, *Living Your Yoga: Finding the Spiritual in Everyday Life* (Berkeley, Calif.: Rodmell Press, 2000), p. 61.

Good Health (page 140)
Brother Achalananda, cited in Margaret Wolff, "Whole Health: An Interview with Brother Achalananda," *Yoga International,* October/November 1996, p. 34.

Disharmony and Ill Health (page 141)
Shri Yogendra, cited in Sitadevi Yogendra, *Yoga Physical Education (for Women)* (Bombay, India: The Yoga Institute, 1947), p. 25.

Bodily Surrender (page 141)
Pandit Usharbudh Arya, *Superconscious Meditation* (Honesdale, Pa.: Himalayan International Institute of Yoga Science and Philosophy, 1974, 1978), p. 121.

Sitting Still (page 142)
Vijayendra Pratap, Deborah Willoughby, "Exploring the Inner Side: The Science of Yoga: An Interview with Vijayendra Pratap," *Yoga International,* November/December 1991, p. 31.

Under Your Own Steam (page 142)
Marcia Moore and Mark Douglas, *Diet, Sex, and Yoga* (York, Maine: Arcane Publications, 1966, 1970), p. 65.

The Benefits of Relaxation (page 143)
Tarthang Tulku, *Skillful Means* (Berkeley, Calif.: Dharma Publishing, 1978), p. 19.

Be Like a Tree (page 143)
Lizelle Reymond, *To Live Within* (Baltimore, Md.: Penguin Books, 1973), p. 121.

Antigravity Yoga (page 144)
Vanda Scaravelli, *Awakening the Spine* (New York: HarperSanFrancisco, 1991), p. 115.

ASANA (PAGES 144–45)
B.K.S. Iyengar, *Iyengar: His Life and His Work* (Porthill, Idaho.: Timeless Books, 1987), pp. 496–97.

13. THE BREATH OF LIFE

BREATH IS FOREMOST (PAGE 148)
Brihad-Aranyaka-Upanishad (6.1.1). Translated from the original Sanskrit by Georg Feuerstein.

THE BREATH OF LIFE (PAGE 148)
Kaushitaki-Upanishad (3.2.1). Translated from the original Sanskrit by Georg Feuerstein.

THE BREATH IS THE WATER OF LIFE (PAGE 148)
Donna Farhi, *The Breathing Book* (New York: Henry Holt and Company, 1996), p. 13.

BECOME A VESSEL FOR LIFE (PAGE 149)
Donna Farhi, *The Breathing Book* (New York: Henry Holt and Company, 1996), p. 5.

INHALING ENERGY (PAGE 150)
Vimala Thakar, *Life as Yoga* (Delhi, India: Motilal Banarsidass, 1977), p. 94.

BREATHING AS CONSCIOUS PRACTICE (PAGE 150)
Tenzin Wangyal Rinpoche, *The Tibetan Yogas of Dream and Sleep* (Ithaca, N.Y.: Snow Lion Publications, 1998), p. 135.

TRUE BREATH CONTROL (PAGE 151)
Laghu-Avadhuta-Upanishad (2). Translated from the original Sanskrit by Georg Feuerstein.

THE WAVE OF THE BREATH (PAGE 151)
Swami Veda Bharati, *Therapy as Transcendental Science* (Rishikesh, India: Sadhana Mandir Trust, 1998), p. 382.

MINDFUL BREATHING (PAGE 152)
Henepola Gunaratana, "Taming a Wild Elephant," in *Breath Sweeps Mind: A First Guide to Meditation Practice*, ed. by Jean Smith (New York: Riverhead Books, 1998), pp. 155–56.

Flow (PAGE 152)

Stephen Cope, *Yoga and the Quest for the True Self* (New York/London: Bantam Books, 1999), pp. 248–49.

Relaxing with the Breath (PAGE 153)

Rolk Sovik, "Watching the Mind Watching the Breath," *Yoga International,* August/September 1997, pp. 43, 45.

Breathing Away Fear (PAGE 154)

Jean Klein, *Be Who You Are* (London and Dulverton, England: Watkins, 1978), p. 44.

14. LOVE, SEX, AND BEYOND

Love Is Radiance (PAGE 158)

Bubba Free John (Adi Da), *The Paradox of Instruction* (San Francisco: Dawn Horse Press, 1977), pp. 86–87.

Love and Happiness (PAGE 158)

Maharishi Mahesh Yogi, *Transcendental Meditation* (New York: The New American Library, 1963), p. 284.

Love Is Blind (PAGE 159)

Sri Ramakrishna, cited in Lex Hixon, *Meetings with Ramakrishna* (Boston, Mass.: Shambhala Publications, 1992), p. 98.

Love Is All There Is (PAGE 159)

Jean Klein, *Neither This Nor That I Am* (London and Dulverton, England: Watkins Publishing, 1981), p. 40.

The Cradle of Love (PAGE 159)

Swami Sivananda Radha, *Mantras: Words of Power* (Porthill, Idaho: Timeless, 1980), p. 22.

The Reciprocity of Love (PAGE 160)

Stephan Bodian, *Meditation for Dummies* (Foster City, Calif.: IDG Books, 1999), p. 158.

Boundless Love (PAGE 160)

"Mahatma" M. K. Gandhi, *The Mind of Mahatma Gandhi,* ed. by R. K. Prabhu and U. R. Rao (Ahmedabad, India: Navajivan Publishing House, 1967), p. 202.

THE LAW OF LOVE (PAGE 161)

Swami Rama, *Inspired Thoughts of Swami Rama* (Honesdale, Pa.: The Himalayan International Institute of Yoga Science and Philosophy of the U.S.A., 1983), p. 91.

LOVE AND SEX (PAGE 161)

Eknath Easwaran, *Thousand Names of Vishnu* (Petaluma, Calif.: Nilgiri Press, 1987), p. 51.

TRUE LOVE (PAGE 162)

Swami Rama, "Freedom on the Field of Action," *Yoga International*, March/April 1992, p. 21.

IGNITING LOVE (PAGE 163)

Bhole Prabhu, "Bhakti Yoga: Path of Love and Devotion," *Yoga International*, January/February 1992, p. 30.

DEVOTION (PAGE 163)

Shankara, *Shivananda-Lahari* (76). Translated from the original Sanskrit by Georg Feuerstein.

WHO LOVES THE LORD? (PAGE 164)

Sri Ramakrishna, Swami Nikhilananda, *The Gospel of Sri Ramakrishna* (New York: Ramakrishna-Vivekananda Center, 1952), p. 137.

TRUE LOVE TRANSFORMS (PAGE 164)

Swami Chetanananda, *Dynamic Stillness: Part Two: The Practice of Trika Yoga* (Cambridge, Mass.: Rudra Press, 1990), p. 190.

RISING ABOVE SEX (PAGE 165)

Swami Chidananda, *The Philosophy, Psychology and Practice of Yoga* (Distr. Tehri Garhwal, India: The Divine Life Society, 1984), p. 216.

THE LANGUAGE OF LOVE (PAGE 165)

Swami Rama, *The Art of Joyful Living* (Honesdale, Pa.: Himalayan International Institute of Yoga Science and Philosophy, 1989).

LOVE AND NONATTACHMENT (PAGE 166)

Swami Vivekananda, *Karma-Yoga and Bhakti-Yoga* (New York: Ramakrishna-Vivekananda Center, 1982), pp. 39–40.

CHASTE LOVE (PAGE 166)

Lewis Thompson, *Mirror to the Light: Reflections on Consciousness and Experience*, ed. by Richard Lannoy (London: Coventure, 1984), p. 102.

15. GREAT REALIZATIONS IN SMALL THINGS

LIVING YOGA (PAGE 170)

Sri Aurobindo, *The Synthesis of Yoga* (Pondicherry: Sri Aurobindo Ashram, 1976), p. 2.

LIBERATION NOW (PAGE 170)

B.K.S. Iyengar, *Iyengar: His Life and Work* (Porthill, Idaho: Timeless Books, 1987), p. 520.

TRUTH IS HERE (PAGE 170)

Dogen, trans. by Thomas Cleary and cited in *Breath Sweeps Mind: A First Guide to Meditation Practice*, ed. by Jean Smith (New York: Riverhead Books, 1998), p. 37.

CONTENTMENT (PAGE 171)

Satguru Sivaya Subramaniyaswami, "Who Do You Think You Are?" *Hinduism Today,* May 1999, p. 10.

OPENNESS (PAGE 171)

Swami Chetanananda, *Dynamic Stillness: Part Two: The Fulfillment of Trika Yoga* (Cambridge, Mass.: Rudra Press, 1990), p. 101.

EMBRACING LIFE (PAGE 172)

Lizelle Reymond, *To Live Within* (Baltimore, Md.: Penguin Books, 1973), p. 174.

SEEING BEAUTY EVERYWHERE (PAGE 172)

Nancy Phelan and Michael Volin, *Yoga for Women* (New York: Harper & Row, 1963), p. 35.

BATHING IN BEAUTY (PAGE 172)

Hari Prasad Shastri, *Self-Knowledge* (London: Shanti Sadan, Winter 1989), p. 29.

TASTING THE SWEETNESS IN EVERYTHING (PAGE 173)

Swami Chidvilasananda, *The Yoga of Discipline* (South Fallsburg, N.Y.: SYDA Foundation, 1996), p. 42.

CONVERSING WITH NATURE (PAGE 173)

Swami Sivananda Saraswati, cited in Swami Prembhava Saraswati, "The Power of the Garden," *Yoga* (Sivananda Math: September 1999), p. 27.

THE EYES OF THE SOUL (PAGE 174)
Meher Baba, *Life At Its Best* (New York: Perennial Library, 1972), p. 58.

INSPIRATION (PAGE 174)
Hari Prasad Shastri, *Meditation: Its Theory and Practice,* 9th ed. (London: Shanti Sadan, 1974), p. 11.

ENTHUSIASM, THE SECRET OF ETERNAL YOUTH (PAGE 175)
Swami Bua, age 110, cited in "Quotes & Quips," *Hinduism Today*, May/June 2000, p. 14.

PEACE IS OUR GREATEST GIFT (PAGE 175)
Thynn Thynn, *Living Meditation, Living Insight: The Path of Mindfulness in Daily Life* (Sebastopol, Calif.: Sae Taw Win II Dhamma Center, 1998), p. 36.

SEEING REALITY WITH A CALM MIND (PAGE 176)
Swami Rama, *Inspired Thoughts of Swami Rama* (Honesdale, Pa.: The Himalayan International Institute of Yoga Science and Philosophy of the U.S.A., 1983), p. 121.

SPIRITUAL BLINDNESS (PAGE 176)
Maharaj Charan Singh, *Spiritual Discourses* (Punjab, India: Radha Soami Satsang Beas, 1964), p. 62.

BEYOND STRUGGLE (PAGE 177)
Swami Chetanananda, *The Breath of God* (Cambridge, Mass.: Rudra Press, 1973), p. 287.

PERFECT SILENCE (PAGE 177)
Swami Satyeswarananda Giri, *Babaji: Volume I: The Divine Himalayan Yogi* (San Diego, Calif.: The Sanskrit Classics, 1992), p. 65.

BEING PRESENT (PAGE 178)
Gurani Anjali, *Rtu: Meditational Poems*, abridged ed. (Amityville, N.Y.: Vajra Printing & Publishing, 1995), p. 97.

DEATH IS A BEGINNING (PAGE 178)
Hari Prasad Shastri, *Self-Knowledge* (London: Shanti Sadan, Summer 1992), p. 93.

THE UNIMPORTANCE OF DEATH (PAGE 179)
B.K.S. Iyengar, *The Tree of Yoga* (Boston: Shambhala Publications, 1988), p. 35.

ALL IS BRAHMAN (PAGE 179)
Hari Prasad Shastri, *Self-Knowledge* (London: Shanti Sadan, Spring 1994), p. 71.

DISCOVERING THE SUBTLEST OF THE SUBTLEST (PAGE 180)
Chandogya-Upanishad (6.12.1–3). Translated from the original Sanskrit by Georg Feuerstein.

16. MEDITATION AND PRAYER

THE MIND MACHINE (PAGE 183)
Richard Hittleman, *Guide to Yoga Meditation* (New York: Bantam Books, 1969), pp. 38–39.

BRINGING THE MIND HOME (PAGE 183)
Sogyal Rinpoche, "Bringing the Mind Home," *Breath Sweeps Mind: A First Guide to Meditation Practice,* ed. by Jean Smith (New York: Riverhead Books, 1998), p. 9.

THE MIND IS LIKE A BIRD (PAGE 184)
Hari Prasad Shastri, *Meditation: Its Theory and Practice,* 9th ed. (London: Shanti Sadan, 1974), pp. 22–23.

IMMORTAL MINDFULNESS (PAGE 184)
Nagarjuna, cited in The Venerable Rendawa, Zhon-Nu Lo-Dro, *Nagarjuna's Letter,* trans. by Geshe Lobsang Tharching and Artemus B. Engle (Dharamsala, India: Library of Tibetan Works & Archives, 1979), p. 47.

THE ARROW OF ONE-POINTED THOUGHT (PAGE 185)
Maharishi Mahesh Yogi, *Transcendental Meditation* (New York: The New American Library, 1963), p. 138.

THE POWER OF CONCENTRATION (PAGE 185)
Tarthang Tulku, *Skillful Means* (Berkeley, Calif.: Dharma Publishing, 1978), p. 29.

ONE-POINTED MIND (PAGE 186)
Brahmacharini Nitya, "Living Your Practice: Meditation in Action," *Yoga International,* November/December 1992, p. 17.

SURFING MEDITATION (PAGE 187)
Stephan Bodian, *Meditation for Dummies* (Foster City, Calif.: IDG Books, 1999), pp. 148–49.

DON'T TRY (PAGE 187)

Pandit Usharbudh Arya, *Superconscious Meditation* (Honesdale, Pa.: Himalayan International Institute of Yoga Science and Philosophy, 1974, 1978), p. 76.

WATCHING THE WATCHER (PAGE 188)

Rudolph M. Ballentine, "Uncovering the Unconscious," *Yoga International*, December/January 1998, p. 26.

MEDITATION IS DRILLING (PAGE 189)

Eknath Easwaran, *Thousand Names of Vishnu* (Petaluma, Calif.: Nilgiri Press, 1987), p. 42.

WORSHIPPING IN THE TEMPLE OF THE BODY (PAGE 190)

J. Donald Walters (Swami Kriyananda), *Do It NOW!* (Nevada City, Calif.: Crystal Clarity, 1995), p. 23.

MEDITATION IS NO KALEIDOSCOPE (PAGE 190)

Swami Rama, *The Art of Joyful Living* (Honesdale, Pa.: Himalayan International Institute of Yoga Science and Philosophy, 1989), p. 17.

TRUTH ALONE (PAGE 191)

Sri Chinmoy, *Yoga and the Spiritual Life* (Jamaica, N.Y.: Aum Publications, 1974), p. 25.

MEDITATION AND FREEDOM (PAGE 191)

Jiddu Krishnamurti, *Five Conversations* (Beckenham, England: Krishnamurti Foundation Trust Ltd., 1968), p. 16.

A PORTABLE PARADISE (PAGE 192)

Paramahansa Yogananda, *Sayings of Yogananda* (Los Angeles: Self-Realization Fellowship, 1968), p. 90.

UNITING THOUGHT AND ACTION (PAGE 192)

Ernest Wood, *Concentration: A Practical Course* (Benares, India/Chicago: Theosophical Publishing House, 1913), p. 19.

MEDITATION AND LIFE (PAGE 192)

Pandit Usharbudh Arya, *Superconscious Meditation* (Honesdale, Pa.: Himalayan International Institute of Yoga Science and Philosophy, 1974, 1978), p. 77.

17. FREEDOM AND HAPPINESS

THE MANY FORMS OF FREEDOM (PAGE 195)
Swami Vivekananda, *Karma-Yoga and Bhakti-Yoga* (New York: Ramakrishna-Vivekananda Center, 1982), p. 101.

TOWARD INNER FREEDOM (PAGE 196)
Swami Avyaktananda, *Letters to a Truth-Seeker* (London: The Vedanta Movement, 1943), pp. 9–10.

ASLEEP, AWAKE, ENLIGHTENED (PAGE 197)
Richard Hittleman, *Guide to Yoga Meditation* (New York: Bantam Books, 1969), pp. 63–64.

DISCOVERING THE HIGHER SELF (PAGE 198)
Chandogya-Upanishad (8.7.1). Translated from the original Sanskrit by Georg Feuerstein.

SELF'S LUMINOSITY (PAGE 198)
Hari Prasad Shastri, *Self-Knowledge* (London: Shanti Sadan, Spring 1992), p. 61.

INNER SUNRISE (PAGE 199)
Swami Muktananda, *Secret of the Siddhas,* trans. by Swami Chidvilasananda (South Fallsburg, N.Y.: SYDA Foundation, 1980), p. 61.

DAWNING OF THE INNER LIGHT (PAGE 199)
Swami Nityananda, *Voice of the Self* (Balaji Nagar, India: P. Ramanath Pai, 1962), p. 33.

FREEDOM (PAGE 200)
Tarthang Tulku, *Skillful Means* (Berkeley, Calif.: Dharma Publishing, 1978), p. 3.

HOME, SWEET HOME (PAGE 200)
Swami Jyotir Maya Nanda, *Yoga Quotations from the Wisdom of Swami Jyotir Maya Nanda,* ed. by Swami Lalitananda (Miami, Fla.: International Yoga Society, 1975), p. 200.

SURRENDERING ALL (PAGE 201)
Swami Chetanananda, *Dynamic Stillness: Part Two: The Fulfillment of Trika Yoga* (Cambridge, Mass.: Rudra Press, 1990), p. 275.

THE LUTE OF THE BODY (PAGE 201)
Vimala Thakar, *Life as Yoga* (Delhi, India: Motilal Banarsidass, 1977), p. 270.

SOUL'S MUSIC (PAGE 202)
Swami Jyotir Maya Nanda, *Yoga Quotations from the Wisdom of Swami Jyotir Maya Nanda,* ed. by Swami Lalitananda (Miami, Fla.: International Yoga Society, 1975), p. 229.

INFINITY (PAGE 202)
Sri Ramakrishna, cited in "M.," *The Gospel of Ramakrishna,* revised edition by Swami Abhedananda (New York: Vedanta Society, 1947), pp. 421–22.

I AM NEITHER THIS NOR THAT (PAGE 203)
Avadhuta-Gita (1.66–67). Translated from the original Sanskrit by Georg Feuerstein.

THE FINAL ACCOUNT (PAGE 203)
Meher Baba, *Life At Its Best* (New York: Perennial Library, 1972), p. 82.

ABOUT THE AUTHOR

GEORG FEUERSTEIN, Ph.D., is the founder-president of Yoga Research and Education Center (*YREC*), a nonprofit organization in Sebastopol, California. He has authored numerous books, including *The Yoga Tradition, The Shambhala Encyclopedia of Yoga, Tantra,* and *Lucid Waking.*

He also is editor in chief of the *International Journal of Yoga Therapy* and has contributed several entries to the *Encyclopedia of Religion,* in addition to serving on the editorial board of the in-progress multivolume *Encyclopedia of Hinduism.* He regularly gives talks and seminars on Yoga philosophy, history, and literature tailored to promote the yogic discipline of study as an integral aspect of Yoga practice.

Georg has studied and practiced Yoga from a young age and has dedicated his life to the preservation of authentic yogic teachings. He can be contacted at: Yoga Research and Education Center, 2400A County Center Drive, Santa Rosa, CA 95403 or by e-mail at mail@yrec.org.

Sustainable Society
Hazel Henderson
Beyond Globalization

HAZEL HENDERSON. Com

Firmly Rooted
Sprout up
grow - assert art